Advance praise for

Reflecting on Autoethnographic & Phenomenological Experiences: A Caregiver's Journey

"In *Reflecting on Autoethnographic & Phenomenological Experiences: A Caregiver's Journey*, Donald R. Collins has created a powerful and important research volume on an unbelievably difficult topic as he shares his experiences as a caregiver for his wife. Both researchers and caregivers will benefit from the sharing as the book is a profound teaching tool for those who attempt, and even need, to combine their very personal life and circumstances with their professional research. This combination and the life support and solace it can provide is literally the most important reason to read this volume. Further, the sharing is both intimate and difficult, yet provides life affirming experiences and perspectives for all of us."

—Gaile S. Cannella, Independent Scholar
Former Professor Texas A&M University-College Station, Arizona State University-Tempe, and Velma Schmidt Endowed Chairperson, University of North Texas

"As a caregiver of parents with Alzheimer's and scholar, I found *Reflecting on Autoethnographic & Phenomenological Experiences: A Caregiver's Journey* to be a remarkable example of qualitative research methodologies employed in a relatable sense. The author walks the reader through a personal journey as he and his family go from one stage to the next of providing care for their loved one experiencing cognitive memory loss. Its thorough representation of the life of a caregiver is an inspirational must read for medical practitioners, caregivers, and researchers using qualitative methodologies as it provides depth in understanding the changing realities encountered by the author and his children as they manage life and provide care for his wife and their mother in an educational context."

—*Kamala V. Williams, PhD, Manager, Prairie View A & M University*

"Donald Collins's personal account of caring for his wife in *Reflecting on Autoethnographic & Phenomenological Experiences: A Caregiver's Journey* not only chronicles day to day activities but provides interpretations of giving care and what it might mean to his wife. His subjective narrative enlightens clinical nurses, providers, professionals, family, and volunteer caregivers by revealing a glimpse of the attention to intimate detail in caring for his partner. The book is a must read for all caregivers."

—*Linda Deadrick, RN, MSN*

REFLECTING ON AUTOETHNOGRAPHIC & PHENOMENOLOGICAL EXPERIENCES

Exploring Qualitative Inquiry
Gaile S. Cannella, Editor

Exploring Qualitative Inquiry is a subseries within The **Qualitative Inquiry: Critical Ethics, Justice, and Activism** series. The broader critical series is a collection designed to provide a cross-disciplinary overview of the use of qualitative research as an avenue for justice and critical transformative activism/action socially, environmentally, and related to more-than-human/human entanglements. This type of work often engages philosophically with emergent, and often marginalized, approaches. The subseries is a set of shorter volumes, each designed to introduce a philosophical frame, component, and/or methodology put forward by a particular critical research scholar. Upon introducing the basic perspective and frame, each volume also provides an example research study to illustrate the particular view.

Exploring Data Production in Motion
by Teija Rantala (2019)

Exploring Deleuze's Philosophy of Difference
by David Bright (2020)

*Reflecting on Autoethnographic & Phenomenological Experiences:
A Caregiver's Journey*
by Donald R. Collins (2021)

Gaile S. Canella (EdD, University of Georgia) is an independent scholar who has served as a tenured full professor at Texas A&M University–College Station and at Arizona State University–Tempe, as well as the Velma Schmidt Endowed Chair of Education at the University of North Texas. The editor of the Qualitative Inquiry: Critical Ethics, Justice, and Activism series is interested in reviewing manuscripts and proposals for possible publication in the series. Scholars who wish to be considered should email their proposals, along with two sample chapters and current CVs, to the editor. For instructions and advice on preparing a prospectus, please refer to the Myers Education Press website at http://myersedpress.com/sites/stylus/MEP/Docs/Prospectus%20Guidelines%20MEP.pdf. You can send your material to:

Gaile S. Cannella
gaile.cannella@gmail.com

REFLECTING ON AUTOETHNOGRAPHIC & PHENOMENOLOGICAL EXPERIENCES

• • • • • • • • • •

A Caregiver's Journey

BY DONALD R. COLLINS

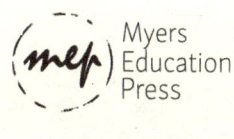

GORHAM, MAINE

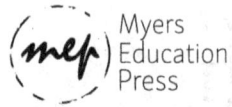

Copyright © 2021 | Myers Education Press, LLC

Published by Myers Education Press, LLC
P.O. Box 424 Gorham, ME 04038

All rights reserved. No part of this book may be reprinted or reproduced in any form or by any electronic, mechanical, or other means, now known or hereafter invented, including photocopying, recording, and information storage and retrieval, without permission in writing from the publisher.

Myers Education Press is an academic publisher specializing in books, e-books, and digital content in the field of education. All of our books are subjected to a rigorous peer review process and produced in compliance with the standards of the Council on Library and Information Resources.

Library of Congress Cataloging-in-Publication Data available from Library of Congress.

13-digit ISBN 978-1-9755-0339-0 (paperback)
13-digit ISBN 978-1-9755-0338-3 (hardcover)
13-digit ISBN 978-1-9755-0340-6 (library networkable e-edition)
13-digit ISBN 978-1-9755-0341-3 (consumer e-edition)

Printed in the United States of America.

All first editions printed on acid-free paper that meets the American National Standards Institute Z39-48 standard.

Books published by Myers Education Press may be purchased at special quantity discount rates for groups, workshops, training organizations, and classroom usage. Please call our customer service department at 1-800-232-0223 for details.

Cover design by Teresa LaGrange

Visit us on the web at **www.myersedpress.com** to browse our complete list of titles.

*I dedicate this book to my wife, the love of my life;
to our beautiful daughter, my rock;
and the memory of our beloved beautiful son, Cody* †.

Disclaimer: *The information in this book is not intended or implied to be a substitute for professional medical advice, diagnosis, treatment, or care. The author makes no representation and assumes no responsibility for the applicability of information contained in this book. You are encouraged to seek and review all information contained in this book regarding any medical condition or treatment with your physician.*

Contents

Prologue: Remembering
xiii

Chapter 1
Introducing a Caregiver Researcher's Life
1

Chapter 2
Ethics and Moral Considerations
29

Chapter 3
From Caring to Caregiving
49

Chapter 4
Mixing Critical Qualitative Methods:
Autoethnography and Phenomenology
77

Chapter 5
Safely and Softly Up and Down the Staircase and Axiology
103

Epilogue
127

About the Author
129

Index
131

Acknowledgments

First and foremost, I would like to thank my Lord and Savior Jesus Christ with whom all things are possible! Next, I thank my wife for her devotion to me. Although I wish I did not have the content for such a work, she is my inspiration and the greatest blessing in my life. She is my living spirit. Our daughter has been my rock for her unyielding and selfless attention, devotion, and care of her mother. Her genuine and persistent concern for me is so beyond words. Our beloved Cody is my inspiration, and he and his loving kindness are always in my thoughts. I acknowledge our parents for what they taught us and the values they instilled in us. I thank my brothers, Carlton Collins, Artis Collins, and Troy Collins, and our only dear sister, Linda Collins Deadrick, for being there. I also thank all other family and friends for their devotion and support. In particular, I am ingratiated with our niece, LaKesha Collins, for her faithfulness to my wife. She has taken such good care of her, and I thank you.

I would like to thank my series editor, Gaile Cannella, for her generous time, thoughts, and constructive feedback on this endeavor. I am thankful to you as my teacher, mentor, encourager, and colleague. I am beholden to Stephanie Gabaree for her superior copyediting skills that prepared my manuscript for its final publication. I am appreciative of Chris Myers as publisher for his vision and patience. I feel honored to know you. Thanks to the team at the Myers Education Press for all of your support.

Without the support of my Prairie View A&M University family, I could not have completed this book. Thank you, friends and colleagues.

Finally, I thank my circle of medical support that gives me hope.

Prologue: Remembering

Early Reflections From My Journal and Memory

My wife getting lost for most of the day grabbed my attention. Two to three times a week, she visited her elderly father, who lived about twenty miles away. She left our house midmorning and, by 3:00 p.m., had not returned. This was not uncommon, but a little after 2:30 p.m., she told me she was preparing to come back home. Around 5:00 p.m., she told me she was on her way home but was in traffic. I remember thinking that I wished she had left earlier because in Houston traffic started jamming up around 3:00 p.m. At 6:00, I called her again, but she did not pick up. I called her dad and he informed me that my wife left a while ago. I asked our son and then our daughter if they had heard from their mother, and both stated that she was at their grandfather's house. I asked them both to try to reach her on her cell phone. Seven o'clock passed. Both of our children informed me they could not reach their mother and said they would call others and keep trying to reach her. I tried to brush concern aside and told them she probably stopped to shop. Our son quipped aloud that his mom did not like to shop unless one of them needed something. I had thoughts about that statement but left it alone. Plus, I could tell our son was starting to worry too. I obsessively called her phone and tried not to panic. I began planning where I would start looking for her and how to ask our children to help me without causing them to panic like I was starting to. A little after 8 p.m., my wife came through our back door and was visibly shaken. I asked her why she didn't answer her phone, and she told me she had gotten lost. This was alarming to me because my wife had always navigated Houston with ease. I hugged her to calm her and asked what happened, which she struggled to remember.

My heartbreak was overwhelming because I believed I should have picked up on what was going on. The heartbreak was mixed with guilt because my wife's sister told me that something was going on with her memory and suggested she should go to a doctor. Around this time, a friend of my wife's also told me she noticed my wife having problems with her memory. In each case, I was unsure of what they were talking about. Also around this time, my wife continued to drive and carry on what appeared to be her normal activities of daily living—except something was off. She made our bed less often, and eventually, she stopped making the bed. I assumed she had just gotten too busy. But making the bed was something she usually did because she said it made our bedroom look neat, even when it might need tidying up. She wasn't tidying up like she insisted on doing daily. I was oblivious to much of her change in behavior as I never assumed anything like dementia was happening to my sharp and intelligent wife. One of the reasons I believe I did not notice her impaired memory and judgment was because my wife was a fastidious note maker. I first noticed her note making as early as high school but paid attention to it on a visit home when I lived out of town before we were married. She made "to do" work notes. I was intrigued with her note making in a little worn calendar she kept in her purse. She maintained her social calendar there too, like when I came home and we went out. Since we were just best friends, I was impressed she put my name and the duration of my visit in her calendar. Of course, she had church and family happenings along with work notes. She told me her "secretary" maintained her work calendar. After we married and went on vacations, she would record down to the penny our spending. This would annoy me, as my system was to budget events, days, and weeks and then to just go home when the money ran out. But my wife knew the details of our vacation spending. Nonetheless, I hoped that I could nurse my wife back, but intellectually, I knew that unless there was a hormonal issue, this would not be the case.

Chapter 1

• • • • • • • • •

Introducing a Caregiver Researcher's Life

> *To everything there is a season, and a time to every purpose under the heaven:*
>
> *A time to be born, and a time to die; a time to plant, and a time to pluck up that which is planted;*
>
> *A time to kill, and a time to heal; a time to break down, and a time to build up;*
>
> *A time to weep, and a time to laugh; a time to mourn, and a time to dance...*
>
> ECCLESIASTES 3:1–4, KJV

Introduction: Thinking Myself

I wrote this book to explore and reflect on my caregiver journey with my wife as she experiences the season and the daily effects of early-onset *frontal temporal dementia* (FTD). This chronicle is viewed through the lens of autoethnography and phenomenology. The issue of dementia is highly personal and overwhelming to the individual experiencing it and their family. Dementia, while uninvited, was the logical diagnosis of my wife's life struggles in this season. It has become obvious a fight on this front was unwinnable. And it is a fight that is leaving scars on all our family members. Rather than give in, however, I decided to win on another front. I decided that I would be active in figuring out how to care for my wife and give her the best quality of life I could. I decided I would function in the here and now, not throw away our dreams but alter their outcomes.

God, faith, and religion have always been present in my life to different degrees. I was born into a believing family. My grandmother, "Granny," attended the Church of God in Christ (COGIC). For two summers, when I was about 12 years old, my younger brother and I stayed with my grandmother in a town that was about 80 miles southwest of Houston in the county where my mom grew up. My mom grew up in an area called Cedar

Lane, Texas, on a farm her family owned. After my maternal grandfather died, my grandmother moved to the city. This was after my mother had finished college, married my dad, and begun having children. Next to faith, education was important to my grandmother and her children. During these summers, my mother went to Abilene Christian College (a university now) to obtain teaching endorsements, and my older brother stayed with my father during the week, visiting us on the weekends. I can think of fewer special times in my life than these summers because we got to live with Granny and our two aunts who were still in high school. We had the run of her house, and it seemed, except on at least two occasions (lighting matches in a closet and making an international call), that we did no wrong. There was nobody Granny did not know. And most of them worshiped with her. Many were relatives, and at some point, many migrated from the country to the small city. Granny and all these new people had ties to the country church Granny attended before she moved to the city. My only recollection of the country church was at my grandfather's funeral, during which one of my mother's friends held me too tight during the entire service. Even though I did not recognize it at the time, Granny's network in the city reported on everywhere my brother and I went, and that party line was a real phenomenon in the city and in the country when we went. Granny, through her quiet and sweet demeanor, made each of her grandchildren feel special. It was more that her demeanor was the relationship she had with God, and she was always leading us in prayer, reading scriptures to us, and telling us how good God could be. Sunday worship services and the many evening services were active with loud church music and preaching that seemed to go on forever. There were several things we could not do in her sight, including playing cards or marbles on her porch or property because this was the devil's work. We always found a place to do this until her network told her and we had to move to another location. Hiding and being found out was part of the intrigue in our young play lives.

My mother raised us in the Church of Christ (COC). Although I am not certain, I believe my mother grew up in COGIC but converted to COC during her college years. From what I understand, my mother converted several of her family to COC. COC is similar to COGIC in that we believe in the sanctification of baptism. Although there are many other doctrinal differences, the most noticeable difference is the absence of

INTRODUCING A CAREGIVER RESEARCHER'S LIFE

musical instruments in the COC. I must confess that I have not always been proud of my belief—not that it was not a faith to be proud of, but as a youth, I was embarrassed by it because it was like being a "mama's boy." But I always complied with my parents' demands of conforming to church doctrine, attendance, and activities. Although not always faithful, the church provided me with all the resources I needed during my most difficult times. Under the tutelage of the church and my parents, I developed a relationship with my Lord and Savior that spans my entire existence. Along with my parents, I was almost in junior high school before I learned that my father grew up Methodist. Although I was intrigued by this, my father supported the religious doctrine of the COC.

I learned to read in the church when I was 5 years old, in Sunday School. I was taught to read from the first 11 verses of the Beatitudes, Matthew 5. Even though my parents read to me up to and beyond this time and our home being rich in print with the *Ebony* and *Jet* magazines, the *Houston Chronicle* and the *Houston Forward Times*, calendars, encyclopedias, and other print media, I was not compelled to read until my Sunday School teacher presented each child a verse to read. Although I do not remember which verse I read, I remember it being one of the first few verses because after the teacher introduced the lesson of Jesus going to the "Mount" to teach the multitudes, she told us that each of us would read a verse and proceeded to start the "read-aloud" process. Because I was on the first row (and I was one of the first to arrive at the room), I would be one of the first to read. I remember practicing so that I could perform my reading part. The two children before me seemed to read with great ease, and it was my turn too soon. My first attempt to read was a disaster and I felt embarrassed. The teacher had to tell me each word. And because of this, I kept reading my verse over and over again and did not pay attention to those who read after me. I found out later that others had struggled as much as I had. At the end, the teacher read the verses, and I paid more attention to her rereading so I could read the verse as well as possible the next time. Even though I made a point not to sit on the front row, to avoid being one of the first to read in Sunday school, it seemed I was always called on to read a scripture verse.

When I told my mother about my reading struggle and that I needed to learn to read, she seemed too encouraging, wanting to practice reading right then. She told me not to worry because I would learn to read well in first grade. Of all my teachers, my first-grade teacher was my favorite; she taught me to read and introduced me to my favorite food, French fries.

Growing up, our lives were centered on church. Most of my mother's friends were connected to church in one way or another. We attended church on Sunday mornings and evenings and on Wednesday nights for Bible study. Because people came from all over Houston, our church started zone meetings on what I remember to be other nights. My mother attended our zone's meetings and other zones' meetings when we were out and about. Vacation Bible School (VBS) was an experience because of the great fellowship and, of course, the punch and cookies always served afterward.

When we became older, possibly around sixth grade, my older brother and I were picked up by men from the church who lived near us to attend the men's training classes and other activities like baseball practice. We were taught how to conduct ourselves as Christian men. Specifically, this involved performing expected roles during church services, such as serving communion, taking up the offering, ushering, and the like. I remember asking when I should put my offering in the tray and being told that because we (men) were role models for the church, I should put it at the front of the entire church. The discussions were always interesting because they primarily focused on how to behave as a man in church and in our communities. Many other lessons occurred such as biblical stewardship for the earth's resources. I was fascinated to learn of this immense responsibility. Some of these teachings coincided with my sixth-grade year when we learned about conservation and a political push on this topic. Embedded in this particular focus was also a push to keep our local community and world environments clean by picking up trash, conserving water, and being proud of our neighborhoods.

After seeing a baptism when I was 8 years old, I began asking questions and soon after asked to be baptized. At the beginning of high school, we started attending youth ministry gathering at White churches. These gatherings reminded me of VBS during my youth. However, there was a difference as we burst through puberty into adolescence, with the weight of integration's desegregation segregation. Refreshments were basically the same as VBS. Black and White adolescent males talked over these refreshments and made plans to see each other the next time, while few of the White girls ever spent much time with us.

Prayer was ordinary in our home. I saw most of the adults in my extended family and friends pray. Whenever a prayer was being offered, out of reverence, everyone was expected to stop any movement and bow their heads until it ended and almost everyone said amen. It seemed rooted in their souls. Sometimes their praying looked similar, like when my father blessed our family meals when we ate them together. These were the prayers we heard them say. Before the children led prayers, I heard both pray for our family and its safety and for wisdom and direction, prosperity, and protection against hurt, harm, or danger. Their praying could look different too. I saw my parents say little prayers throughout the day. But it was my father's daily prayer rituals that left a lasting impression on me. Any time I was in my father's presence when he got out of or got ready for bed, he would get on his knees at the edge of my parents' bed and pray. I do not remember when I noticed it, but he seemed serious and unwavering from this whispered ritual. As young children, I remember seeing him before bed, running to him for attention and asking him what he was doing. He would tell us he was praying. Eventually, we asked him what he was praying about, and he would always tell us he was praying about us. Sometimes he would stop praying to attend to us, or as we got older, he would tell us to pray with him, as he prayed aloud. Although not aware of it at the time, when I look back, these were times during which my father had solace and fervently talked to God. All in all, I am confident that our parents' prayers protected or got my siblings and me through or kept us from harm, hurt, or danger. Prayer is the most important legacy my parents gave to me. While I am aware that different caregivers and researchers pull their strengths from different sources, my relationship with God grounds me and gives me the strength to face any obstacle. No matter what is troubling me, when I pray, I know I can turn it over to God and He will get me through it. I pray constantly for guidance and patience as a caregiver.

Philosophical Perspectives

Several broad lenses were applied in the unfolding of this book. These represent interpretive beliefs I hold in my academic and personal lived experiences and are constantly evolving. They all reflect social behavioral engagements and observations. While these lenses reflect contextual glimpses of my positions in autoethnography and phenomenology focusing on caregiving, they are by no means exhaustive.

Philosophical Methodological Lens

Critical Theory. Critical theory originates from 1923 (Jeffries, 2017) from a study group (Horkheimer, 1982). With funding from Felix Weil, the Institute for Social Research, also known as the Frankfurt School at the University of Frankfurt, Germany, was created to denounce the scientific method as a means to explain the oppression of marginalized people (Padmanabhan, 2006). The assembled leading Marxist scholars included Max Horkheimer (1895–1973), Theodor Adorno (1903–1969), Herbert Marcuse (1898–1979), Walter Benjamin (1892–1940), Fredrich Pollock (1894–1970), Leo Lowenthal (1900–1993), Erich Fromm (1900–1980), Franz Neumann (1900–1954), and Jürgen Habermas (1929-), (Corradetti, 2021; Jeffries, 2017). The institute was forced to close in 1933 by the Nazis and subsequently moved to New York City at Columbia University, where it became known for "critical theory." The move to the United States marked a move from idealism to pragmatism, although the latter still mirroring the former in many ways (Bohman, 2019; Horkheimer, 1982). Early Frankfurt School critical theorists distinguished the philosophy from traditional theory in seeking an "emancipation from slavery" (Bohman, 2019, p. 1) in a general reference to freedom for all humans from dominion and subjugation of the powerful, thereby seeking to effect social change. Traditional theory sought truth that can be identified and described. Critical theory seeks to explore perceived truths by turning them inside out to discover multiple human realities (Horkheimer, 1982). An important distinction between the Frankfurt School and subsequent theories is that the former uses "Critical Theory" as a proper noun, hence its capitalization. This distinction refers to the assiduous work and thinking of the Frankfurt School. The latter, "critical theory," is used as an adjective, in which an attribute has been ascribed to a noun to modify or describe it. Critical Theory extends to "ethics, political philosophy, and the philosophy of history" (Bohman, 2019, p. 1).

While critical theory espouses Marxism and a big umbrella of emancipation, it is unclear who this manumission included at its inception, with its founders, and subsequent leaders, being all German men. Western Marxism, however, viewed capitalism as the singular (Marcuse, 1964) cause of "human suffering and social misery" (Rabaka, 2006, p. 748). W. E. B. Du Bois (1868–1963) and other Negro[1] scholars, such as the economist

---
1 *Negro* is used in historical context.

Abram Lincoln Harris (1899–1963) and Carter G. Woodson (1875–1950) (Kendi, 2017), perceived the cause of human suffering and social misery to be caused by White racism. Despite Marx declaring that "labor in a white skin can never be free as long as labor in a black skin is branded" (Kendi, 2017, p. 335), Du Bois, Woodson, Harris, and Black antiracists and assimilationists believed that Marx did not view racism to be a dominant issue of the social ills experienced by Blacks in the United States.

Critical theory is often thought of as emanating from the Frankfurt School with an emphasis on condemning capitalism as the cause for oppression. However, its major feature of "critical thought" has allowed the emergence of critical race theory, dis/ability critical race theory, and Black feminist theory. These theories intersect during my caregiving experiences.

Critical Race Theory. This book searches phenomena in autoethnographic experiences that make them redolent. Through a critical race theory (CRT) and critical qualitative inquiry or a critical inquiry lens, the primary phenomenon of caregiving as lifesaving and maintaining is examined for an emergent narrative. The most offensive experiences for me as a man growing up in the southern city of Houston, Texas, are the evils of racism. In Richard Delgado and Jean Stefancic's (2012) primer *Critical Race Theory*, the authors espouse that racism permeates all of society and is "ordinary" (p. 7). This major "tenet" is a shocking reality for Black and people of color. It is not an accepted reality but one, nonetheless. It is how White privilege (Diangelo, 2018; Wise, 2011) is carried out and who carries it out in society. Racism is based on hegemonic power that is, today, subtler but just as dangerous ever. Delgado and Stefancic postulate CRT as a "movement . . . of activists and scholars interested in studying and transforming the relationship among race, racism, and power" (2012, p. 3). Critical race theory questions "liberal order" (Delgado & Stefancic, 2012, p. 3) and its by-products of partiality that are biased against people of color.

Because of progressive laws and social norms, historical overt racism has become more subtle. Its intractable forms are less obvious when employed through microaggressions. They are retractable because racist views may be covered by a generative or "prosocial" (McAdams & Hart, 1998) façade hiding the racist's true worldview of racial superiority.

As a critical qualitative inquiry, positive aspects (Lloyd, 2016; Yu, 2018) of caregiving are explored. Specifically, Yu (2018, p. 24) delineates these as "personal accomplishment and gratification, feelings of mutuality in a dyadic relationship, increased family cohesion and functionality, and a sense of personal growth and purpose in life," with features of spiritual faith. Furthermore, as indicated throughout this book, the lived experience is imbued as a caregiver journey through the season of life situated in my wife's lived experience with dementia. Important is the focus on the benefits of spousal caregiving with moral capacity (Gyekye, 2011) rather than feelings of burdening. I believe this is achieved by my seeking and maintaining a "positive spiritual perspective" (Quinn, Clare, & Woods, 2012, as cited in Yu et al., 2018, p. 23) and mindset. This narrative is further explored for meaning to the individual, personal, and subjective interpretations of lived experiences.

Key Framework Terms and Underlining Suppositions

Key terms are elaborated throughout the book in each chapter. Initially, the following working terms are presented: *Autoethnography* refers to the introspective. *Axiological suppositions* refer to insider values and biases that shape the narrative. *Critical qualitative inquiry* refers to complex lived experiences with meanings on multiple and nuanced levels of analysis throughout this book. *Ontological suppositions* refer to complex lived realities and their meanings. *Phenomenology* refers to the exploration of an experience with insider status.

The explored phenomenon of caregiver for this book is composed of multiple dimensions and layers. The outer layer is qualitative research. The next layer is autoethnography. The third layer is phenomenology. As the third layer is inspected, experiences of a redefined role, loss, grief, agony, and bereavement are revealed. This essence is of an insider's lingering personal experience of the agony in loss of a loved one's personhood.

Becoming Aware of Autoethnography

I became aware of autoethnography when I first attended the International Congress of Qualitative Inquiry (ICQI). My first encounter was overshadowed by my "deer in the headlights" experience with the breadth of the assemblages of qualitative inquiries on display. Most memorable to me at this first encounter was a dance performance to the beat of drums. Interestingly, I was drawn to the session by a paper on narrative analysis. When the performance began, I looked around the full room to plan my exit. But, by the end of the performance analysis, I had greatly expanded my knowledge of what qualitative inquiry offered not only to qualitative study in academia but also on subjective reflections. I gained an appreciation of different and interpretive modes of this methodology. Immediately, I realized that even though I had an experience as a musician, I would never be able to emulate the dance execution.

It was not until my second attendance of a preconference workshop led by Norman Denzin at the ICQI that I encountered autoethnography. Besides the session being led by one of the preeminent scholars in autoethnography, I resumed my interest in what made this inquiry research. From this point on, I began to study and explore autoethnography. Subsequently, a colleague and I attended Carolyn Ellis and Arthur Bochner's session about writing a collaborative autoethnography. Along with two other colleagues, we presented a collaborative autoethnography of three college professors. In the paper, we explored intersections of our narratives, careers, aspirations and professional microaggressions. Our analysis revealed individual career paths with achievement, determination, and persistence, but were plagued with racism and sexism.

Encountering Phenomenology

I encountered phenomenology in my graduate coursework and considered it as I explored approaches for my dissertation. Ultimately, I decided on grounded theory for my dissertation to study the education of African Americans in the southern Texas region. But I maintained an interest in first person experiences of subjects in cultural settings. Over the years, I have presented papers on this approach and served on several dissertation committees where students focused on phenomenology.

Prior to learning about autoethnography, I was introduced and limited to biographies such as Anne Frank, Hellen Keller, and J. F. Kennedy during my K-16 schooling. In graduate school my exposure became more balanced and I was drawn to historical Black biographies that included, but were not limited to, James Baldwin, Fannie Lou Hamer, Langston Hughes, Zora Neale Hurston, Martin Luther King, Harriet Tubman, Ida B. Wells, Sojourner Truth, Jackie Robinson, Malcolm X, Ray Charles, Stevie Wonder, Neil Diamond, Michael Jackson, and many others. Postdoctorate, I was enamored with biographies in ethics, such as Henrietta Lacks and the men of the Tuskegee Syphilis Study. Reading these and other biographies, over the years, led me to read eye-opening racial and political autobiographies such as *Narrative of the Life of Frederick Douglass, an American Slave* by Frederick Douglass, *Up from Slavery* by Booker T. Washington, *Bone Black: Memories of Girlhood* by bell hooks, *Nigger* by Dick Gregory, *Malcolm X* by Alex Haley and Malcolm X, and *Black Boy* by Richard Wright. Exploration of multiculturalism and ethnography along with biography and autobiography guided me to develop an interest in autoethnography.

Moving Into Context: Thinking With My Journal

As my wife's caregiver, I seek to provide a comfortable quality of life, as she experiences moderate early onset frontotemporal dementia (FTD). The caregiver role is complex and multidimensional. Daily living care requires thinking and acting for my loved one whose cognition has diminished to the point of requiring constant care. The myriad of daily tasks drain me emotionally, not only because of the total care delivered to my loved one, but because as the disease has progressed, not only has her cognition deteriorated, but her language ability has declined, from the time of her diagnosis, from slightly impaired verbal expression, to a diminished ability to articulate to near total loss of speech. This near total loss of speech makes it difficult for her to receive and generate speech. Moreover, she is no longer able to comprehend written and spoken language. While she is sometimes able to emit responses to short questions, her communication is distorted. For example, when she needs to use the bathroom, she says "...it hurts in my house." Or, she may say, "I want to go home." At which I comfort her with touch and assure her that she is safe. This latter phrase has multiple meanings. It can mean she is uncomfortable and anxious. Or, it could mean she wants to go the bathroom.

I constantly pray for and am blessed with patience and renewal every morning from God. This patience helps me to help my wife. I help my wife slowly stand up from her recliner in our living room, wait, help her to stabilize her body and then slowly lead her to step, then walk, then turn left, walk, and then turn right, and then to walk to the bathroom door. When we are near the door, she stops walking because she senses the flooring is about to change from a dark to a light color and because the walls change from a light to a darker color and I've not turned on the bathroom light. Darkness in the bathroom increases her anxiety. But I encourage her to resume walking to the threshold of the door. Sometimes she walks over the threshold, but when she is trying to comprehend the changes in flooring and lighting, she pauses until I gently pull her by both hands across the threshold and into the bathroom. Once we are fully in the bathroom, I ask her if she is "ok." Sometimes she answers, "Yes," but on many other occasions, she says "Yes" thinking I am calling her name. Her name sounds like "ok." I change my question to, "Are you alright?" She is distracted in the bathroom by a large mirror. When she turns to look into it, she thinks her reflection is another person. When this phenomenon first emerged, we covered the mirror with butcher paper because she would argue with her reflection. At first, this was troubling, but as I adjusted to her confusion with her reflection, I joke, "You are prettier than her." She laughs and seems to know that my statement does not make sense.

Preview: Merging Phenomenology into Autoethnography

The narrative in this book emerges from the infusion of one substantive approach into the overarching substantive approach and compels the researcher to consider the impact of each. The autoethnographic overarching approach is itself a complex mixture of approaches that represent legitimate bodies of research. The merged approaches are exploratory in nature. In the present mixed approach, phenomenological elements focus more on introspection consciousness than on the other main character, my wife. Methodological overlapping concepts include as listed by Janice M. Morse (2017) and detailed by Max van Manen (2014), reflective, descriptive, interpretive, and engaging endeavors. Self-analysis and heart-searching seek a deeper spiritual understanding rather than a day-to-day temporal existence. While temporal tasks such as constantly cooking, cleaning, bathing, and etcetera are important, at the deeper level there is meaning to the whole lived experience. A question that arises is what does this phenomenon of husband caregiver mean in autoethnography as participant and researcher? The essence of the meaning is based on subjective reflections.

The frame of autoethnography supports the emergence of multiple personal caregiver perspectives that were explored through the use of life story narrative, autoethnography, and autobiography. In the life story autobiographies, the subject and author's reflections on journaling reflect value in caregiving. The autoethnography perspective is one in which the primary subject provides personal self-reflection to meanings in the family milieu. The strategy of constant comparison of reflections and observations provides further autoethnographic introspection. This consciousness seeks to explore the meaning of a phenomenon revealed within the context of a particular setting. Reflective journals and observations seek to understand if and how shared experiences transcend multiple contexts. The inquiry further seeks to objectively distinguish what is expressed, expected, and what is not expressed. Subjectively, the inquiry seeks introspective connections between reflections and life experiences.

Meanings

Viktor Frankl's (1959, 2006) *Man's Search for Meaning* revealed his suffering as a prisoner in Nazi concentration camps during World War II. Meaning in Frankl's account displays how the quintessence of survival requires being purely spiritual and devoid of earthly possessions. Spiritual survival of suffering (Gregg, 2016) is an ordinary consequence of immense pain, trauma, loss, or grief. Finding meaning clarifies our purpose by our choosing how we cope with our dilemma. As a spouse caregiver, meaning is the realization that the cared-for is my greatest gift from God, His favor, and this devalues all acquired material belongings. Through spiritual survival, extraneous matters are pushed aside or even off the table so that my attention is singularly focused on what matters: God and my family. In realizing how vulnerable life is and understanding how quickly things can change, this means I must be there for my wife because she deserves my love and attention. The coldness of the disease of dementia is warmed not only by the care I am able to shower on my wife but also by the knowledge that I am providing life-sustaining attention to her.

Broadly, multiple practical insights emerge from the caregiver husband's constant reflections and these are positioned throughout this book. More specifically, however, pragmatic (Sullivan, 2001) meanings include monitoring my voice tone, slowing my physical guidance "way" down, completely finishing one behavior before starting another, and valuing

INTRODUCING A CAREGIVER RESEARCHER'S LIFE

singular focus ability. Each person experiences dementia differently. The reciprocal experience between wife and husband carer defines the essence and reality (ontology) of caregiving.

Meanings from the present research are constructed from four basic paradigms (Creswell & Poth, 2018) that include the reality of the phenomenon (caregiving) under scrutiny (ontology), knowledge (epistemology) of the phenomenon (caregiving for a loved one with dementia), critical consciousness (axiology), and the research procedure (methodology). These paradigms are presented in various forms throughout this book. Separately, each of these constructions has a singular meaning. At their intersection, the constructions transform into new didactic complex meanings. The intersection of epistemology and axiology, for example, in autoethnography offers unique opportunities for interpretation and meaning.

The subjective intersection of caregiving for dementia (epistemology) and critical consciousness (axiology) in caregiving fosters behaviors and mindsets conducive to the well-being of my life partner. Behaviorally, this juncture is reflected in a culture of care or theorized in the 1950s as care culture (Leininger & McFarland, 2002). While Leininger and McFarland (2002) posits that although the care culture is positioned in the nursing profession, it offers important ideals for non-nursing family caregivers who value providing practical, quality care to loved ones. These ideals include "holistic and multidimensional" care that were highlighted during the 1960s' term "ethnonursing" (Leininger & McFarland, 2002, p. 190). Leininger's focus on culture in nursing care present similarities to ethnography specifically and to autoethnography (as examined later) generally. Built-in components of the care culture include non-nursing family caregiving consistent with understanding the ethnic, family, religious, and community dynamics. Moreover, another component of the theory is the expectation by family caregivers that professional nursing (and other medical) practitioners value the same dynamics.

Characters: Embodied and Remembered

He who finds a wife finds what is good and receives favor from the LORD.
PROVERBS: 18:22 NIV

Jesus . . . said . . . ,"Truly, truly, I say to you, you will weep and lament, but the world will rejoice. You will be sorrowful, but your sorrow will turn into joy."
JOHN 16:19–20, ESV

Biographical Reflections

My wife and I grew up in a large metropolitan area in the state of Texas and attended public school from kindergarten until high school graduation. I attended segregated schools through the sixth grade and desegregated schools from seventh through 12th grade. My wife attended segregated schools through fourth grade and desegregated schools from fifth grade through her high school graduation. My wife attended a public university, and I attended a small private liberal arts college in Texas. My mother and my wife's mother were transferred to White schools during desegregation. We both accompanied our mothers to their respective desegregated schools. We grew up in different Black neighborhoods and attended the same White high school we transferred to.

I met my wife when we were in eighth grade. My mother visited my wife's parents' home one day with me and my siblings. From what I gathered, my wife's mother and my mother met in a university class they took together. After their visit, my mother drove to the cul-de-sac to turn around. As we drove back down the street, my older brother and I noticed several girls talking to each other in front of one of the girl's houses. I recall making eye contact with one of the girls. In 10th grade, I recognized a girl who was also trying out for the marching band and finally remembered seeing her 2 years before when my mother drove down her street. Over the next weeks, she and I talked, and one day in a calm voice, she accused me of going into her room, picking her clarinet up from her bed, and playing it. She told me that this happened one summer when I visited her house with my mother. Although I could not articulate my thoughts, I felt accused of crossing a boundary I would not cross. In a fussy but quiet tone, she went on to tell me she had to change her reed and wash the mouthpiece. Confused, I told her I did not play her clarinet when we visited her house, but I remembered seeing it on her bed when I went to the bathroom. I told her I remembered seeing her down her street. Hurt, I walked away. That night I found out that my older brother had been the culprit. A day or so later, this girl came over to me and started a conversation. It would be years before I told her my brother had played her clarinet. By then, she and I had become best friends. When she was not with her boyfriend, we spent time together. After college, we became romantically involved and married.

Seven years after marrying my best friend, we welcomed our daughter into our family. Two years later, we welcomed our son into the world. My wife was so happy mothering our children. In a clairvoyant way, she had told me she had seen the faces of our children in a dream. Before we married, my wife told me her dream was to have six boys. I remember being speechless.

My wife wrote across genres. She enjoyed poetry as well as prose. Sometimes her poems gave me shivers when she explained them to me. I realized her poems had depth and that she put in the time to achieve the voice and effect she desired. Still, I was not drawn to poetry. My wife has a master's in technical writing. She earned it when she worked as the director of the Patient Simulation Program at one of the University of Texas Medical Branch campuses. But she loved creative writing, and sometimes her creativity went over my head. She liked artsy kind of writing and things. I am reminded of one of her doctoral classes. Although I do not remember the exact paper assignment, I remember her paper. When she finished the paper, she asked me to read it. I remember thinking it was in the typical format: cover sheet, title page, references, and so on. But I was astonished when I turned to the first text page. The text was written in a vertical line from the top to bottom of the page, with commas, periods, colons, and other punctuation. About three quarters down the page, a horizontal row intersected with the vertical line of words. Multiple vertical lines of words intercepting multiple horizontal rows filled the remaining pages. I did not know what to say. I knew two things: First, it was her art. Second, I knew I could not criticize her paper because I did not understand it enough to interpret it. It reminded me of poetry. I cautiously asked her if her paper was a form of creative writing. She to me no and that it was an analysis. I felt paralyzed because I could not bring myself to read the words down the vertical line and then the intercepting row. Nervously, I asked her to read the paper to me. When she read the paper to me, I felt better. But I asked her if she should write the paper in the more traditional way. She discarded my veiled recommendation and told me the professor wanted a creative paper. When she explained it to me, I recognized the analysis with the interceptions and other positioning having meaning. Nevertheless, it was an over-the-top paper. Her professor loved, loved, loved her paper when she presented it to the class. And, when she received comments and feedback, accolades filled the page showing her professor's admiration for what my wife had created.

I, on the other hand, did not have much affinity for creative writing and none for poetry. As an English teacher, interpreting and writing poetry were part of the curriculum, and I taught them effectively. Technically, I understood poetry enough to teach and demonstrate how to interpret and write poems. Likewise, I was always pleased, as a teacher is when he knows he contributed to his students' growth, when my students found their voice in poetry and produced meaningful verse.

As I sat to make notes on this book, I had a poetic experience in which the following poem flowed from me. I was surprised because, as I stated, poetry was not something I enjoyed writing. This poem is a narrative free verse that I allowed to emerge. It was an emotional release that gave me gratification and an appreciation of poetry I lacked. It is a poem of personal sorrow and hope. It is my first poem.

I Remember...
When Dementia wasn't, and
when Cody was.
When we first saw each other, and,
when we met again in high school.
When we were best friends in high school,
and college.
When you would drive me home across town after school.
When my infatuation with you dominated...
When we went to different universities.
When romance entered our lives, and
we dated and got married.
When you tried to tell me what to do.
One of your tests.
When we first argued, and
I couldn't go to sleep, because

I could not be angry with you and sleep, but
we forgave.
When we dreamed about our lives with children, a house, and
growing old together.
When you made me give you money I'd saved for a sprinkler system,
because you said, unbeknownst to me,
we were saving for drapes in our new house.
When our daughter was born, and
then Cody.
When you convinced me I did not need an expensive truck, and
I convinced you we did not need a luxury car, and
we acquiesced because we did.
I know...
That this is all of God's plan.
That your dementia is...
That the most important thing is caring for you,
like you cared for me.

My Wife's Parents. My wife's mother retired as an elementary school teacher. Her father retired as a postal worker. Both worked in their respective careers for over 30 years. They both graduated from Prairie View A&M University with degrees in elementary education and history education, respectively.

My wife's mother. My wife's mother was born in a small East Texas town from where her parents moved to the Houston area. She was slender and about 5 feet 8 inches tall. Her skin tone was like paper-bag brown in color. She enjoyed all types of sports and enjoyed playing basketball in high school. She grew up with three brothers and two sisters. While her sisters remained in the South, two of her brothers moved to Flint, Michigan, during the Great Migration of Blacks from the U.S. South to the North (Wilkerson, 2011). My wife and her mother often reminisced about their musical talent in playing the trumpet.

My wife's mother graduated from Prairie View A&M University with a bachelor's degree in elementary education. She earned her master's degree in school administration from Texas Southern University. I remember my wife's mother telling me she aspired to become a journalist. However, as was a custom when she went to college, her father told her she would be a teacher. That is what she became and taught in the Houston Independent School District for 32 years. But before she began her teaching career, she worked at the *Houston Informer*, a daily newspaper. She was the first in her family to receive a college degree. She was a staunch advocate for education and encouraged anyone she encountered to be lifelong learners.

My wife's mother was married to my wife's father for 51 years. They raised my wife and her younger sister and enjoyed spending time with their extended families. She and her husband were active in the United Methodist Church for 51 years. My wife's mother was active in many social and church roles.

My wife's father. Like his wife, my wife's father was born in a small town north of Houston. His mother and father had three children. One sibling died at an early age. My wife told me that before she and I met, her dad's brother died of cancer. She told me her dad stopped smoking "cold turkey" when his beloved brother died.

My wife's father was slightly over 6 feet tall and lean. He was dark brown, and my wife always described her dad as handsome. He was a warm and quiet man. He grew up in the Houston area with his mother and father. He graduated from the famed Jack Yates High School. My wife told me her dad and mom met at Prairie View A&M University. He graduated with a bachelor's degree in history. He planned to teach but worked for the U.S. Postal Service for more than 30 years.

His large yard was always immaculate, as was his home his wife kept. Although he was a genteel man, he preferred to manage his yard himself. The few times I cut his grass, he jokingly told me my lines were not straight. While we bantered about the straightness of the grass lines, I knew he did not want to relinquish the responsibility to me or anyone else. When he was offered a riding lawnmower, he declined, saying that they did not cut the grass with the precision of a push mower. It was always obvious to me that he doted over his daughters, often calling them by a nickname he had given them.

My Parents. When I began to hear before attending college and read in college that most Black families were led by single mothers, I was perplexed because that was neither my story, nor what I saw in my Black neighborhood. Although I knew families that did not have two parents, this was the exception and rarely did a parent's absence result in an aberration. As a child, I saw things by looking up at my parents with adoration.

As I grew and became a parent, I appreciate the parenting road map of many turns they gave me. And while we were far from being or even looking like the "Brady Bunch," my parents did what parents do, give to and love us unconditionally.

My Mother. My mother also graduated from Prairie View A&M University with a bachelor's degree in home economics. She earned her master's degree at a university in New York. She was the first in her family to graduate from college, with her four younger sisters following in her path. As a young boy, I remember asking her why her older brother did not go to college. She told me he worked so that she and her sisters could go to college. When I first heard the story, I was struck with a child's bewilderment that, over the years, turned into awe of his sacrifice. Even though I did not grasp the concept of money at the time, I was shocked when my mother told me that when she graduated from high school as the valedictorian, her country community awarded her a $50 tuition scholarship. During college, my mom told that me to earn spending money, she cleaned houses and did hair. When she finished college, she was hired as an extension agent, going into communities and homes to demonstrate cooking, cleaning, and other home economics activities. My brothers and I fantasized that she had worked as a secret agent like the ones we saw on the television. Her home extension agent job moved her to a town north of Houston, and this is where she met my father, who worked as a mechanic at a gas station and filled her car with gasoline.

My mother was fair-skinned, about 5 feet 8 inches or so. She was beautiful. For me, my mother's love was the foundation of my understanding of love. When I asked her where I came from, she told me that I was a blessing from God. I was a mother's boy, but so were my brothers. Our baby sister was our parents' crown. When she was born, my parents intimated that with her, they were satisfied with the blessings of four boys and one girl. We were collectively nurtured and connected to our mother in individual ways. My first recollection of my mother was of her cooking in the kitchen. My collective descriptive memory of my mother would be loving, supportive, encourager, teacher, disciplinarian, intellectual, explorer, Christian, protector, and nonviolent advocate. I say nonviolent advocate because my mother regaled being peaceful. She insisted on our best behavior at school, in church, and in our community. Most of the time we complied, and when we did not, we were not in her presence. On one occasion, I remember my mother talking to my brothers and me about not getting into fights. My mother was doing laundry in our kitchen, as that is where our washer and dryer were back then. When we asked her what we were supposed to do if another boy hit us, she said do nothing. It seems like we bombarded her with questions all at the same time. She just said, "Do nothing." At my young age, I remembered learning in Sunday school that Jesus said to turn the other cheek, and I was skeptical about that. I stayed with my mother after my brothers left because her advice didn't seem right to me. As my mom and I talked, my dad came into the kitchen and started making himself a sandwich, hearing the end of the conversation. When my mom left, my dad whispered to me that I should defend myself and with that permission, I did when I needed to.

Sometimes, I wondered if my mother's attention to her children was my reason for articulating early on that I did not want children. Being swept up in her care for us made what she did look like it was easy and supposed to be. My mother seemed to always be willing to take us on an adventure, even if it was just accompanying her to one of her university courses. We were always involved in something and going somewhere. She spent a lot of her time taking me to violin, then piano, and clarinet lessons. In junior high school, I learned to play the bassoon because my band director asked me to. I remember hearing the band director tell my mother that I might be able to get a scholarship to college for the instrument, and I did receive one for a couple of years. So, through high school on many Saturdays, I took lessons for the bassoon. During my last 2 years of high school, I told my parents that I didn't want to take music lessons anymore but wanted to work and spend more time with my friends. Everything had a purpose and a meaning. Sometime at the end of college, I realized that having children required a lot of effort and sacrifice. The constant going was never a problem growing up, but when I had children, I wondered how my mother did so much when my wife and I only had two children compared to my mother and father having five.

My Father. Thoughts of my father are of a handsome brown-skinned man, with a thin mustache. He was probably 5 feet 10 inches, a little taller than I am today. He was lean, strong, and muscular. He worked as a longshoreman and probably loaded and unloaded cargo ships containing heavy bags of grain, coffee, barrels of substances, and the like. When he let me work with him for two of my high school summers, he had been promoted to a heavy machine operator. Having a level of seniority in the Black International Longshore and Warehouse Union, he was able to arrange for me to be near his work area for my first few days. After that, I remember most of the time working with someone who knew my dad. Even though the work was hard, I enjoyed it because I got to hear stories from men I would probably never have heard. The unbridled cursing fascinated me too. And the money was great for a high school student. As I repeated some of the stories to my dad on the way home, he told me not to tell my mother about what I heard, and I fully understood what he meant. When I learned more about the union and asked about joining it, my dad told me I would need to go to college before joining. It was one of those brush-offs parents give their children instead of saying no.

Unlike my mother, my father seemed to like to be at home. I would not go so far as to say he was a "homebody," but it looked as if it was a comfortable place for him. Friends would visit him, or he might visit a close friend in the neighborhood. My dad liked football and watched it on TV as often as he could. We watch football, basketball, and baseball on TV when my dad watched them. From our porch, he watched us play baseball on a church field across from our house, offering tips when he saw we needed them. He took me to Boys Club baseball practices. We took an interest in watching wrestling with him on Friday nights. After finishing our chores or when it was too hot on Saturdays, we watched western movies with our dad. On a night during the week, we gathered in front of the TV to watch *Star Trek* and *Lost in Space*. As we got older, he supervised us mowing the yard, paying particular attention to the lines in the yard and careful edging. Learning this skill came in handy during college to earn pocket money. Saturdays was a day my dad would barbeque. My mom would make the sauce and my dad would grill. One of my younger brothers learned my dad's technique so that his BBQ tastes just like my dad's. I never mastered my dad's technique and would often cause a fire when I attempted to BBQ brisket. My children made fun of me until my brother finally told me to face the brisket fat up.

My father had been married before and had a grown son. I always wondered why my father did not put us in football like he had our half brother. I half-assumed it might have been my mother who discouraged our playing but never got around to asking my parents. My half brother looked like my father and my older brother. Intriguing to me was the fact that I had a half brother, and this made me feel unique. Fascinating to me was the fact that his family was composed of four girls and one boy: the exact opposite of my family. His children were close if not the exact ages of my siblings and me. Being an uncle seemed to be a position of honor for the young boy I was at the time. When I asked my father why he and his first wife divorced, he told me they had married too young.

My father completed sixth grade. His father owned the sole grocery store in the small town where he grew up and met my mom. I remember my dad spending time in his garage maintaining his cars and tools. It was a large tin structure with two large heavy tin doors that could be locked and swung out. During the day, the doors were swung out to let the light in. At night, a single lightbulb illuminated the inside of the structure. The dirt ground floor was where a car could be parked and the raised level was equal in size, spanning the length of the structure, and made of wood. We could not go in there unless he gave us permission. He kept his tools and equipment in there. Growing up I remember seeing a car engine hanging from some structure high in the garage. In the garage, he taught us how to maintain and work on cars. We would go out there and get boxing lessons from my dad. Even though our dad bought my older brother and me a green Gremlin to drive during high school, he made sure it ran without fail. It was not until our friends made fun of the car that we realized how funny it looked. We were just happy to have a car and not have to use one of our parents' vehicles.

My dad was 20 years older than my mother and around the same age as my maternal grandmother. I learned this fact when I asked my mother to see my birth certificate and saw my parents' birthdates. Even though his discipline was harsher than my mom's, it was infrequent. I recall my dad hugging us frequently and teasing us when my older brother and I began to show him less affection as we grew older. My dad expressed great disdain when his children fought. He told us we were blessed to have each other and how alone he felt growing up as an only child.

Because of my parents' difference in age, they sometimes saw the world differently, and sometimes they had similar views. I recall my father's interest in our education. Where he articulated to us the need to make good grades, my mother insisted on good conduct in school. Misbehaving in school was something my mother did not tolerate. When my mother was told I was misbehaving in third grade, she withdrew me from my school, took me across town, and had me placed in her classroom. At the end of the school year, she failed me. I was distraught and begged my father to talk to my mother. I could tell my father was not happy, but he made an effort not to say anything in front of me. As things turned out, my dad told me that I had to change my "conduct" and that if I went to summer school, my mom might allow me to pass to the next grade.

When my older brother and I would complain to our parents about being disciplined at school, my mother would quip that she was sure that if we did not do what we had been accused of, we surely had done something to deserve punishment. My father, on the other hand, would question us to find out if we were indeed innocent. So when I misbehaved in school, I would usually tell my dad so he would be a buffer to my mom's one-sided thinking that teachers were always right. My teacher-mother held other teachers in high regard and seemed to believe whatever she was told about us. I recall a time when a high school teacher called my home and told my dad that I cursed her. When my friend dropped me off at home, my dad was livid with me because the teacher had called and given him her details. He usually got home from work around 3:00 p.m. and usually had dinner waiting for us. I looked forward to his fried biscuits and chicken after school. Although he didn't say it, I got the impression he was waiting for my mom to arrive so that they could talk about the teacher's accusation. When my mom finally arrived home, my discussion with my dad had escalated to him accusing me and me denying it. I kept trying to explain to him that the words I said sounded like what the teacher said but that I had used other words. In his anger, he began to list the things I would not be able to do as punishment. We were going back and forth—him dolling out punishments, me objecting—with our tempers escalating at each of my denials. I kept telling him I would not curse at a teacher. I remember thinking that he looked like he was going to get his belt, but he never did, having ceased that infrequent practice since the beginning of junior high school. Finally, he sent me to my room. Defiantly, I stood still glaring at him and he looked back at me. My mother had been standing outside listening before coming inside. She probably saved me from receiving a blow from my dad's anger. She told me to go to my room and that she would come and talk to me after she talked to my dad. The first thing my mom said to me was that I had to apologize to my father. Even though I knew I had not cursed my teacher, I was surprised when she told me she did not think I said what the teacher accused me of. But then she reminded me that I had been known to use those curse words. So she reasoned with me that the teacher could have made a mistake. And, as my dad had demanded, I would need to apologize to the teacher. I remember thinking, "They've switched on me." Of course, in hindsight, both of my parents would probably say that they would do many things differently. As a child and a teenager, and in the heat of the moments, I felt my parents were often unfair. But my cherished recollections are like the following journal entry I made shortly after my wife was diagnosed with dementia.

> ***Coffee with my daddy.*** *Every day is new, old and the same old same old. I look forward to each morning's cup of gourmet coffee. It is the time I feel close to my late father who rose early to go to work as a longshoreman. Despite his attempts to be quiet, I listened with anticipation for his moving around in the kitchen. But it was the smell of coffee percolating in the metal pot that drew me toward the kitchen. As I stood in the doorway, I waited for him to motion me into his private coffee time and space so I could have five or ten minutes alone with him, not having to share him with my mother, my brothers, and later my little sister. Few words were uttered, but this undivided attention gave me precious memories that are triggered each morning when I make my morning coffee. These memories include me watching him drink his coffee and, as I got older, him giving me the coffee cup saucer to slurp the coffee he spilled.*
>
> *Other memories of my relationship with my father include him whipping and chasing and probably cursing me home at dusk with a switch because he was angry I was not heading home, as he admonished me to do for several weeks. I was winning at the four-square ball game we played when I felt the licks from the switch hit my legs and heard my dad's angry voice that I should be heading home by now. Stuck in those memories are my friends laughing at me. But a few days later reminding me to head home so I would not get in trouble again with my dad. At bedtime, my daddy kissed me on my head, looking into my eyes as to ask, "We good?" Except for being disobedient, it was not until high school that I understood my daddy's discipline that day when I learned about Black boys disappearing in Houston and in the South around that time.*

> *The next morning, I woke up smelling coffee brewing and hearing my dad piddling in the kitchen. I went to the kitchen to have coffee with my dad before he went to work.*
>
> *As I grew older, these early morning intimate moments became fewer and fewer, as I moved into my teenage years distancing from him and completely stopped when my dad died at the end of my junior year in high school.*

When my father died, my older brother and I were told to drive to an aunt's home to meet my mother. I don't remember how we got there and the reason for the request. I recall asking why we needed to travel across town to my aunt's home. In a warm voice, my aunt told me to come to her home. I asked if my mom was alright and was told she was alright but pleaded with me to come and I told her we would come right away. As soon as I got off the phone with my aunt, I immediately called the hospital my dad had been in after suffering a stroke the week before. When I arrived home after school, I entered our home to find my dad's coin collection scattered all over the floor. My mother called home to tell me my dad had a stroke and had been taken to the hospital by his friend. When I asked her which hospital and where it was, she seemed indifferent. I now realize that she was in shock and was trying to keep herself together in this crisis. By the time my brother and I arrived at the hospital, several of my mom and dad's family and friends had arrived. When I was allowed to go into my dad's hospital room, I was struck by my dad's fragile appearance and his eyes. I looked in his eyes and saw a fragility I did not recognize in the father I had always known to be strong and healthy. I remember thinking that I could not recall my dad having even a cold and now he was not able to move any part of his body, except his eyes. He seemed to be talking to me through his eyes to tell me he would be fine. Holding his hand, I told him I would be back to see him soon. I visited him every day with my mom and brothers and sister. Even though we knew people who were ill and experienced medical crises, I had never experienced a crisis so close to me. Throughout the week, my mom spent all her time with my dad at the hospital. My mother was in a place I had never witnessed her in during my life. In a protective effort, her sisters allowed her to seclude herself in a bedroom.

Reader Thought Questions and Further Reading

1. How did you become aware of autoethnography?
2. How did you become aware of phenomenology?
3. Why does Collins propose mixing qualitative methods in this book?

Compare the meaning in Viktor Frankl's (1959, 2006) *Man's Search for Meaning* to the constructed meanings Collins contemplates.

1. Who are the characters in Collins's narrative?
2. What are the personalities of the characters?
3. Do the characters set in the researcher's memory? Why?
4. Must an autoethnographic character be alive? Why or why not?
5. Define *biography*, *autobiography*, and *autoethnography*.
6. What would be the topics of your biography?
7. What would you include in your autoethnography?
8. How successful was the author in merging biography, autobiography, and ethnography to form autoethnography?
9. List the biographies you have read and when you read them. How racially and ethnically diverse were they?

Compare Stephen Butterfield's (1974) *Black Autobiography in America* to Zora Neale Hurston's (1984) *Dust Tracks on a Road: An Autobiography*.

1. How are they similar and different?
2. What did the authors write about?

Read Sherick Hughes's (2020) "My Skin Is Unqualified: An Autoethnography of Black Scholar-Activism for Predominantly White Education."

1. What is the autoethnography about?
2. How is it different and/or similar to other autoethnographies?
3. Create a conceptual map for the theoretical framework provided by the author.

4. Write a conceptual framework for the theoretical framework provided by the author.

References

Bohman, J. (2019, Winter). Critical theory. In E. N. Zalta (Ed.), *The Stanford encyclopedia of philosophy.* https://plato.stanford.edu/archives/win2019/entries/critical-theory/

Butterfield, S. (1974). *Black autobiography in America.* University of Massachusetts Press.

Corradetti, C. (2021). The Frankfurt School and critical theory. In *Internet Encyclopedia of Philosophy.* https://iep.utm.edu/frankfur/

Creswell, J., & Poth, C. N. (2018). *Qualitative inquiry research design* (4th ed.). Sage.

Delgado, R., & Stefancic, J. (2012). *Critical race theory: An introduction* (2nd ed.). New York University Press.

Diangelo, R. (2018). *White fragility: Why it's so hard for White people to talk about racism.* Beacon Press.

Frankl, V. E. (1959, 2006). *Man's Search for Meaning* (I. Lasch, Trans.). Beacon Press.

Gregg, B. H. (2016). *What does the Bible say about suffering?* Intervarsity Press.

Gyekye, K. (2011). African ethics. In E. N. Zalta (Ed.), *The Stanford encyclopedia of philosophy.* https://plato.stanford.edu/archives/fall2011/entries/african-ethics/

Horkheimer, M. (1982). *Critical theory: Selected essays* (M. J. O'Connell, Trans.). Continuum Publishing Corporation.

Hughes, S. (2020). My skin is unqualified: An autoethnography of Black scholar-activism for predominantly White education. *International Journal of Qualitative Studies in Education, 33*(2), 151–165. doi:10.1080/09518398.2019.1681552

Hurston, Z. N. (1984). *Dust tracks on a road: An autobiography.* University of Illinois Press.

Jeffries, S. (2017). *Grand Hotel Abyss: The lives of the Frankfurt School.* Verso.

Kendi, I. X. (2017). *Stamped from the beginning: The definitive history of racist ideas in America.* Bold Type Books.

Leininger, M., & McFarland, M. (2002). *Transcultrual nursing: Concepts, theories, research, and practice* (3rd ed.). McGraw-Hill.

Lloyd, J., Patterson, T., & Muers, J. (2016). The positive aspects of caregiving in dementia: A critical review of the qualitative literature. *The International Journal of Social Research and Practice, 15*(6), 1534–1561.

Marcuse, H. (1964). *One-dimensional man: Studies in the ideology of advanced industrial society.* Beacon.

McAdams, D. P., & Hart, H. M. (1998). Anatomy of generativity. In D. P. McAdams & E. d. S. Aubin (Eds.), *Generativity and adult development: How and why we care for the next generation* (pp. 7-43). American Psychological Association.

Morse, J. M. (2017). *Essentials of qualitatively-driven mixed-method designs*. Routledge.
Padmanabhan, S. (2006). Skepticism, modernity and critical theory by Philip Walsh. New York: Palgrave Macmillan, 2005 [Book review]. *Human Studies, 29*(3), 405–412. http://www.jstor.org/stable/27642763
Rabaka, R. (2006). The souls of Black radical folk: W. E. B. Du Bois, critical social theory, and the state of African studies. *Journal of Black Studies, 36*(5), 732–763.
Sullivan, S. (2001). *Living across and through skins: Transactional bodies, pragmatism, and feminism*. Indiana University Press.
van Manen, M. (2014). *Phenomenology of practice: Meaning-giving methods in phenomenological research and writing*. Routledge.
Wilkerson, I. (2011). *The warmth of other suns: The epic story of America's great migration*. Vintage.
Wise, T. (2011). *White like me* (2nd ed.). Soft Skull Press.
Yu, D. S. F., Sheung-Tak, C., & Wang, J. (2018). Unravelling positive aspects of caregiving in dementia: An integrative review of research literature. *International Journal of Nursing Studies, 79*, 1–26. doi:10.1016/j.ijnurstu.2017.10.008

Chapter 2

Ethics and Moral Considerations

Do not conform to the pattern of this world, but be transformed by the renewing of your mind.

Then you will be able to test and approve what God's will is—his good, pleasing and perfect will.

ROMANS 12:2, NIV

Brief History of Ethics in Institutional Review Board Context

Historically, measures have been attempted to prevent the abuse of subjects in research. The Code of Hammurabi (Teall, 2014), the Hippocratic Oath (Miles, 2005; Winau, 1994), and the records of Celsus (Ferngren, 2017), a physician, are three of the earliest recorded attempts to define experimentation in contrast with the realm of healing. The emergence of the concepts of experimentation and healing led to methods to regulate each of these processes. The institutional review board (IRB; National Commission for the Protection of Human Subjects of Biomedical and Behavioral Research, 1979), an ethics committee, is a product of these nascent attempts. The curiosity of humans and the investigative aspect of research processes have had an interesting relationship at the intersection of morality, societal norms, and ethical dilemmas. Customs and social values influence the principles applied and the practices associated with the involvement of humans as subjects of study. Often, the purpose and desired outcomes have been aligned according to conscience and prevailing laws.

Ethical dilemmas regarding class, gender, ethnicity, race, and origin surface in written records as early as 1st century CE when the Roman physician

Celsus presented comments that the use of criminals as subjects in dangerous experiments was justified if the benefits to the innocents were outweighed (Jonsen, 1984). The concepts of bondage, gender, and privilege have a tightly woven warp in the tapestry of regulated research. An examination of Celsus's records shows Alexandrian physicians performing vivisection on criminals to advance scientific research. A highly charged debate ensued regarding the use of patients for the benefit of knowledge (Jonsen, 1984). Celsus characterized this practice as unconscionable and tantamount to experimentation, in contrast to treatment.

This philosophy has been revisited time and again throughout history, particularly when faced with the decision to use a select population as the experimental group in a life-threatening experiment. The period most often associated with ethics and regulation are the four decades beginning with 1947 and culminating in 1987. In 1947, in the Nuremberg trials, 23 physicians were convicted of war crimes committed under the guise of medical experiments and resulted in the Nuremberg Code. This code defined 10 points for engaging in ethical research with human subjects. In 1967, the World Medical Association published the Declaration of Helsinki, which was revised as the Declaration of Geneva. This declaration established the physician's code of ethics (Anabo et al., 2019).

African American Participation in Research in the United States

The use of slaves, captured and bound as subjects and victims in research, has changed over time from their being involuntary objects of experimentation (Washington, 2006) to becoming seemingly voluntary participants. During slavery, slaves were subjected to live autopsies in medical schools (Harris, 1996). Blacks were used in other studies over the course of time. However, the research that has caused the most distrust of researchers by African Americans was the Tuskegee Study of Untreated Syphilis in the Negro Male (1932–1972). This study was conducted by the U.S. Public Health Service in Macon County, Alabama, and involved 399 African American male subjects and 201 African American male controls. Not only were the participants not informed that they had syphilis, but they were also not provided treatment of penicillin. Subsequently, it is estimated that between 28 and 100 men died because of syphilis. The news that subjects were deceived and denied treatment was reacted to around the world. The global outrage resulted in the creation of the National

Commission for the Protection of Human Subjects of Biomedical and Behavioral Research in the United States to establish a code of ethics for research of human subjects. In 1979, the commission drafted the Belmont Report. This report established three ethical principles for conducting research with human subjects. These principles include respect for person, beneficence, and justice. These principles are foundational in the regulations of human subjects at all public and most private institutions. Although the Tuskegee Study sparked worldwide outrage and resulted in the Belmont Report, many other studies have violated human rights.

Participant vulnerability emerged as a research safeguard in the United States with the creation of the Belmont Report in 1979.

Disclosure in Autoethnography

Shortly after my wife was diagnosed with dementia, I intellectualized, as did my wife, our situation about what the condition would mean for our family. We were confused and somber in terms of what to do and who to share the diagnosis with. I kept reflecting on when we had a miscarriage before having our first child. When the doctor explained to us what happened, I looked at my wife and could see the pain she was trying to hold in. We avoided eye contact because we did not want to break down in the doctor's office, even though I got the impression he encouraged a response because of the warm and tender care he took as he assured us that the miscarriage was nature's way of getting my wife's body ready to carry a fetus full term. These were the most awkward moments I can remember in our marriage at that time because my wife was on the exam table and I sat across and to her right in a chair looking up at her, with the doctor standing and facing both of us. We opted to stay in the exam room. He explained that we needed to schedule a D&C [dilation and curettage]. As the doctor sat down, he explained the procedure to me, as my wife knew what it was. The doctor's tender delivery of the news did not lessen its impact. His bedside manner was impeccably genuine, as he spent extra time in silence with us until he felt we were ready to leave. He told us to go home and take care of each other and that his office would contact us to schedule the D&C. The doctor nurtured my wife through her next successful pregnancy but left his practice right before our delivery to care for his wife who was experiencing terminal cancer.

This new news was surreal, reminding me of the moments more than twenty years ago, except my wife and I were sitting next to each other and I rubbed her hand thinking it would be comforting. Although I'd read the neuropsychological report, I felt the blow of the revelation. Even though the diagnosis was different, it triggered the memory of avoiding eye contact with my wife. But this time, I could feel my wife looking at me and rubbing my arm to console me, as I held back tears and found it hard to talk to the neurologist. Nevertheless, in a warm voice filled with empathy, the doctor told us to get my wife's affairs in order through legal counsel. Once again, the doctor tenderly gave us news that changed our lives, but this time she conveyed that this diagnosis of dementia was uncurable and terminal. I interpreted this to mean the need to prepare for my wife's death. Over the course of time, the doctor explained the changes to expect and those occurring in the moment.

Guiding Ethical Questions

The reader may ask (Douglas & Carless, 2013) questions simular to those posed by Tullis (2013) to focus the ethical ramificaitons of including others in one's personal narrative. My guiding ethical questions include: "What makes this information important when the topic is ethics?" Other questions might include "What can be revealed?" "Is permission needed in autoethnography, in general, and in this project, in particular?" "Who can information be revealed to?" "What depth of information can be revealed?" "What is the benefit of revealing this information?" "How does the writer protect the characters in his autoethnography?" "Are there alternatives to consent in autoethnography?" "Is there presumptive consent?" "Why am I telling my story?" "Who is the audience?" "Do I have an obligation to the audience?" "What should not be revealed?" "Have I discerned the interesting from the germane?" and "Have I adequately described my phenomena?" Tullis (2013) recommends rigorously maintaining "ethical mindfulness" (p. 99). Although similar to Tullis's questions, my set of ethical questions guided and focused me on the caregiver phenomenon I was exploring.

The IRB and Inquiry Safeguards

Initially, I believed my study did not need IRB approval. However, I was not sure if the IRB would view the risk of my main characters and other actors in the same way I did. Nevertheless, I respected the IRB's protective authority in my proposed study and viewed it as necessary in the broader historical frame of reference. Before initiating my project, I formulated my characters. I would be the main character, and my wife and my daughter would be dynamic characters in my autoethnography. Because my autoethnography would spotlight caregiving for my wife, her identity would be obvious to anyone with whom we had a personal and, in some cases, a professional relationship. Other participants were distant from me (doctors) and were clearly at low to no risk of exposure. Merging groups of actors into composite characters (Ellis, 2007) guarded some identities. Even though the IRB informed me I did not need its approval, I created a proximity scheme to explore and ensure confidentiality and to shield the identity of participants. In an effort to maintain an ongoing ethical mindfulness, whenever I introduced a new character in a story, I used the process in the Sample Proximity Schematic (Table 2.1). This schematic displays a sample of treatment for confidentiality. The top row specifies the character or role of an actor; their relationship, proximity, and insider or outsider status to the researcher and the family; and treatment or disguise. I scrutinized the proximity to me or my wife as a consideration in privacy treatment. The relationship and proximity of the participant overlap as family members are treated with pronouns and, in some instances, as composites. Physicians are referred to by their specialty or by the composite "doctor" and pronouns regardless of their field.

Table 2.1. *Sample Proximity Schematic*

Character	Relationship	Proximity: Close/Distant/ Insider/Outsider	Treatment
(First Name)	Wife	Close	Pronoun
(First Name)	Daughter	Close	Pronoun
Sister	Sister	Close	Pronoun
Oldest Brother	Brother	Close	Pronoun, Composite
Younger Brother	Brother	Close	Pronoun, Composite
Neurologist	Doctor	Distant	Pronoun, Composite
Primary Care Physician	Doctor	Distant	Pronoun, Composite
Obstetrician	Doctor	Distant	Pronoun
Internist	Doctor	Distant	Pronoun, Composite
Nurses, Attendant	Nurses	Distant	Pronoun, Composite
Non-Immediate Family Member	Family Member	Close	Pronoun, Composite

Scholars of autoethnography (Andrews, 2017; Tullis, 2013) advise consulting the IRB as ethical practice. Tullis (2013) provides guidance on protections for the self and others when conducting autoethnography. Incorporating guidelines from other scholars of ethical autoethnography, Tullis provides seven useful elucidated guidelines to consider before and during autoethnography. Tullis guides researchers to do the following:

> (1) Do no harm to self or others. (2) Consult your IRB. (3) Get informed consent. (4) Practice process consent and explore the ethics of consequence. (5) Do a member check. (6) Do not present publicly or publish anything you would not show the person mentioned in the text. (7) Do not underestimate the afterlife of a published narrative. (2013, pp. 256–257)

While consulting with the IRB is debated by autoethnographers, many of the dilemmas I indicated previously may not be recognized by the researcher. It may be akin to the foolishness of a medical doctor treating himself. This is not to say that all IRBs have a balanced and knowledgeable review process. I have heard horror stories at other universities. But doing no harm to participants—and even to the autoethnographer—is paramount. Also important is the protection of the institution. For me, the IRB application was a simple process, and the response was swift. Basically, the IRB informed me I did not need its permission as long as I did not use my wife's and my daughter's names. If I planned to use their names, I would have to go through the review process. Initially, I thought using their names would make their characters real and opted to undergo the review. But, after reading some autoethnographies and reconsidering the value of using their names, I decided to exclude their names. If I used their names, I felt confident I would be approved. I felt this way because when I served on the IRB, our goal was to facilitate good ethical research. If the research plan was not ethical, we recommended measures for it to become so. As far as I knew, this was still the case.

The Allure of Autoethnography

The richness of autoethnography is an attractive approach to graduate students. I have advised students to delay conducting emotional autoethnography because of the psychological aspects inherent in such an undertaking. In research classes, I introduce autoethnography for rigor, breadth, and to help students understand the pictures the approach provides through thick description (Lincoln & Guba, 1985). Specifically, in this effort, I introduce autoethnography to students by having them read Ellis's "Maternal Connections" (Bochner & Ellis, 2016, pp. 171–179). The selection does just what it is intended to do; it evokes emotion and paints a contextual picture. As a response, some students articulate a personal connection and express a sincere interest in autoethnography. These students tell me about taking care of loved ones and how Ellis's story put them in that place, as though they were in the moment. When talking with them, I ask them about their stories, research interests, and what they seek to accomplish, and most of them are emotionally latent to the point of causing tears to flow, becoming angry, or expressing another emotion, based on their respective experiences. I suggest they consider counseling to support them if they choose an emotional autoethnographic topic. I express concern when they tell me they have never addressed the issue. Broadly speaking, I tell them that when we engage with an emotionally latent personal phenomenon, we may need to tap into our supports. These supports might include counseling, psychotherapy, and/or psychiatry, depending on the type of emotion our story entails. Autoethnography takes time and emotional space. It requires mindfulness. It can be an emotional process demanding reflection in solitude, and in my case, prayer. It has the potential for healing. Autoethnography takes us to a place. In terms of anger, I stress that characterizing someone as a villain or a saint (Tamas, 2019) creates audience suspicion. This naivete about one-dimensional character development may also limit one's story and reflect on the author as being petty. Without diminishing feelings of hurt and even harm, if autoethnography is sought to address a slight, it may be beneficial to the story's meaning to look at the bigger picture, such as pathologies. In essence, I am cautioning graduate students on the subject of conducting autoethnography unless it is undertaken with the necessary supports. I make it clear that their design or approach is up to them and their chair. Dealing with emotionally latent issues may require attention that takes them away from a timely matriculation through their program. Some of the issues shared with me by students and not previously addressed include (but are not limited to) a parent's suicide when they were a child, physical and sexual abuse, and turbulent relationships. I do tell them that I have read some really good dissertations using the autoethnography approach and that they should read some to see if it fits with their goals. While I discourage graduate students from choosing autoethnography as their dissertation methodology, in qualitative research, dissertation seminar, and dissertation research classes, I do engage students in a positionality exercise in which they write a "mini" autoethnography focusing on biography, autobiography, and ethnography on a research interest. Ultimately, students state this helps them position themselves in their seminal study.

The parameters of ethics in conducting autoethnography require the inquirer to adequately and clearly explore the roles of all participants. This brings to mind the concept of a participant-researcher. The one who is the subject, directing inquiry on themselves and their culture and writing about them, is exercising dominion in the shaping of a story, as well as the readers' perception of unnamed others. How does this induction move toward doing no harm? Not only does the introspection need to understand its impact on others, but it also needs to show personal deliberation of what is disclosed. Inherent in my autoethnography based on reflexivity journaling is the idea that interpretations from my experiences have been written as text. Personal published disclosure of my personal phenomena cannot be retracted. So careful consideration is paramount about others and to me.

Risks and Vulnerabilities

Power vulnerability has historically been the primary factor in hegemonic research abuse. Historically, minorities, the poor, and the sick, although underrepresented in research, suffered abuse, deceit, and neglect in research. Prior to the Belmont Report in 1979, the treatment of research subjects and participants depended on the moral sensitivity of the researchers. Or was maltreatment at the hands of the researcher the evil of the time?

Washington (2006), in her book, provides historical and comprehensive accounts of moral, unethical, and cruel lapses in the medical care and research African Americans receive across areas that include access, treatment, and follow-up. Washington documents the occurrence of "painful, risky experimental surgery, dosed with radiation and singled out for experiments aimed at finding brain abnormalities linked to violence" (Grady, 2007) on slaves. This practice continued after the emancipation of slaves. Additionally, Washington further provides accounts of denying anesthesia to Blacks because of the myth that Blacks have a higher tolerance of pain. Although, in many cases, researchers and medical providers claim not to intentionally practice bad medicine, apathy and neglect are too often experienced by patients. Regardless, this amounts to immoral medical and ethical racism.

In light of the Belmont Report (1978), the Tuskegee Syphilis Study (1932–1972), and the Henrietta Lacks (1920–1951) story, ethical concerns pose challenges that have to be addressed by researchers of African American respondents in a neoliberal (Fisher, 2007) power and privatization-driven (Rubinstein & Medeiros, 2014) environment. Henrietta Lacks was a bigger than life story (Skloot, 2011) because she has been immortalized through her cancer cells. Without her consent, and through objectification, her cells (known as HeLa) were cultivated by George Otto Gey for medical research and treatment. Neither Lacks nor her family have been compensated for her contribution to science.

Furthermore, scholars in the academy may recognize that trust and suspicion (Gamble, 1997) are major issues faced by researchers of African American subjects in light of the dark deception perpetrated by the medical profession on Black men and families. Despite this knowledge and protections today, neoliberal decisions pose risks that may serve to eradicate earlier protections. In spite of historical moral and ethical lapses, the concept of participant vulnerability did not emerge as a research safeguard in the United States until the advent of the Belmont Report in 1979.

Personal Vulnerabilities

As I reflect on personal vulnerabilities, I am reminded of April Chatham-Carpenter's (2010) article "'Do Thyself No Harm': Protecting Ourselves as Autoethnographer." Her writings persist through personal "triggers" that autoethnography reveals of her "on-going" tensions (Chatham-Carpenter, 2010) with anorexia and embodying the public image of an academic. I find helpful her list of strategies she proposes to protect the "self" when writing. These include making choices about our evocative stories; researching others, controlling the writing while controlling her anorexia, performing personae, and making choices about protecting others (Chatham-Carpenter, 2010). Managing the tensions that pose risks and vulnerabilities in evocative writing is an imperative, particularly when obstacles and triggers are evident.

The biggest vulnerability for me in autoethnography is the ongoing post-trauma-like reactions. Black men learn as youth to deny hurt and not reveal their feelings to the public and even to those close to them. This repression is a protective shield against a racist society as I navigate it daily. Paul Laurence Dunbar's (1895) poem "We Wear the Mask" speaks to not only to collective experiences of the racist subjugation of African American men but also to vulnerability. Dunbar's title and refrain acknowledge the instinct to hide hurt of any kind as doing so is to place myself in an extremely vulnerable position. Even though Dunbar implies that we should remove the mask, he understands its protective features. The mask was always worn or at the ready, except when I was in the presence of my wife. I'm not sure when I began to take it off with her, but by the time we married, I didn't feel the need to wear it in her presence. The only other person I felt this open with was a handful of my closest family and friends. But sometimes I wore it in the presence of my parents to protect them from feeling my hurt. In retrospect, they may have assumed what was really a feigned maturity. And I knew they were wise because they always had a solution to any problem I experienced, even if I rejected them.

Exploring and Arriving at Consent

In autoethnography, the writer must decide how vulnerable to make themselves and remember that what is not said has power too. Sophie Tamas (2019) posits that experiences surrounded with ethical concerns should be thoroughly explored as an ethical treatment. By this treatment, nuances, complexities, and projected consequences (Tullis, 2013) may be revealed for meaning, relevance, and growth.

Constant dilemmas I faced when I decided to write about my journey with my wife's season of dementia were, Would she have consented if she were able to? How would I know if she wanted me to reveal information about her? Although she was physically available, the dementia had rendered her consent unavailable. I believed she would want me to tell our story and how we maneuvered it. The most I could hope for in terms of pure consent as defined in the literature would be retrospective consent (Tullis, 2013, p. 249). It was not explicitly there. But, based on our relationship, I believe I could assume presumptive consent. By the time I began analyzing my journals for retrospection on life, family, and

ETHICS AND MORAL CONSIDERATIONS

relationship, she could not give verbal or written consent. In an effort to triangulate my journal entries, my memory, my focused guiding ethical questions, Tullis's guiding questions, and Tamas's exploration treatment of ethical concerns, I believe I could presume consent.

Familial Aspects of Caregiving

Soon after her diagnosis, my wife and I talked often about how our lives would change and what it meant. She stressed three concerns. First, when I asked her if and when we should let people know, she told me in a soft voice that she wanted to tell people herself. Because of their close relationship, she wanted to tell her father alone. We had lost her mother several years before. Next, she told her sister. She then allowed me to tell my close relatives. She told me she did not want to hide the diagnosis, but just didn't want many people to know until she was ready to tell them or she was not able to. She agreed I could tell my siblings, eventually disclosing it to her aunt and cousins. By then, our daughter, son, or I transported my wife everywhere, so we were included in some of her conversations with others. Her disclosure to friends was very interesting to me. She seems to know just when to tell them. After church one Sunday, I overheard my wife tell a friend to remind her because of "the dementia." I soon noticed she would disclose her diagnosis when a friend told her about a future event she wanted to attend. I was not sure how people interpreted this and told her saying it like that sounded like a joke. She told me to follow up with her friends to let them know about her diagnosis. A few of her friends expressed concern at her disclosure. They wanted to know what they could do. What was surprising was some of her other friends seemed indifferent, not in an uncaring way, but treating her the same as they had before she told them. By now, I had become overprotective and usually hovered near her whenever we were in public.

Second, my wife asked me to make sure that she always looked good. She told me to make sure I dressed her nicely, as she had always done for herself. By this she meant that her clothes matched and fit. Most of the time I have met her request, but on occasion, our daughter has chastised me by saying, "What do you have my mommy in?" But these failures have been few. My wife and I laughed when she told me to watch what our daughter bought for her and put her in. She said she might dress her in young-adult type of dress. I will see if this is edited out of this manuscript when our daughter reads it. Much of the advice online and in print on dressing people who experience dementia suggests loose-fitting attire.

The third request my wife made of me was that her hair look good. At the time we talked about this, I gave it little thought. But the first time I had to take care of her hair; the only beautician I knew my wife liked was an hour away. I suspected salons she frequented were closer to us but did not know their locations. So, for a few years, our daylong trek took us across town to a lady who took excellent care of my wife both styling and just making sure she was safe. Even though this woman was great, I was relieved when a co-worker referred us to an excellent beautician fifteen minutes from our house.

Soon after receiving the diagnosis and when my wife was ready, we told our children. After we talked, I gave them each a pamphlet, which neither of them looked at, and both left on the table. I felt like I was guiding them through a fog I could not see through myself. Their resistance was their way of denial, and I understood. They had close mother–daughter and mother–son relationships. Our lives were slowly, but consistently changing and its focus became ensuring their mother's and my wife's safety, diet, grooming, and all of her activities of daily living. We talked about safety while trying to maintain a high level of independence. Our son, who began practicing and teaching yoga, told us that all his mother needed to do was to get on a yoga schedule and throw away her medication. While he was serious about this, he was diligent in reminding or giving his mother her medication. Nonetheless, he stressed his confidence she could be cured without medication. In subsequent conversations with him, I explained to him the progression of the disease. He began to see his mother's diminished cognition and also became more attentive to her new and unique needs. He cooked and cared for her. He monitored her safety, walked with her, and took her on her errands. He chose jobs at assisted-living communities where he could attend to the needs of the elderly and told us with excitement about conversations he had with residents who also experienced dementia.

He became interested in sketch art and enrolled in college as an art major. Our son was growing up. We took him to week, then monthlong meditation retreats in Texas. He took his first flight alone to Arizona for a monthlong yoga retreat and training. He told us to quit calling him because he was fine. He wanted to go to Asia because of his interest in wanting to travel the world.

Similar to our son's behavior, our daughter did not accept her mother's diagnosis well. I don't know if our daughter had more difficulty with the impending change of her mother, but her resistance to the diagnosis was evident. In spite of joking about our daughter dressing her mother, her behavioral pathology could have been a yearning for her mother to be like she was. Our daughter would often watch her mother as she struggled with her memory, detachment from situations and more and more her flattening affect. Our daughter, like our son and me, never imagined this would happen, but it had, and her well-being became our new reality. I could see she did not know how to deal with her mother's diminishing cognitive ability. Sometimes she seemed robotic in her interactions with her mother, careful not to hurt her. While it was painful for me to see her avoid her mom, I understood and tried to give her space to grow and mature in our ever-changing reality. She struggled with her mother looking fine and being healthy, but her not being fine and the dual ultimate outcomes of her mother's cognitive and physical mortality. My heart hurt as I watched her struggle and grieve at the loss of her mother. As I did with our son, I talked to her about what to expect as the dementia progressed. But her countenance was of defeat for some time and I could see her fear of what would come. Shortly after the diagnosis, my wife and I informed our children that we had given them our medical powers of attorney and their roles. We reminded them of the locations of our last will and testaments and that our daughter had, under an administrator, our durable POA [power of attorney]. My wife and I joked about our son asking us for our bank codes a year before. So, for practical reasons, we told him we would wait for him to be older before adding him as an administrator. Halfway through the explanation of the document to them, I could see tears in our daughter's eyes. Our son was distant but seemed to be listening. When I asked them if they were alright, our son nodded he was, but our daughter moaned, "No," and stood up and walked away. I tried to tell her it was alright. But she had become distraught. It was inconceivable that her mother was losing her cognitive function, her memory, and her life. As time passed, our daughter worked to spend time with her mother, helping her with everything as the dementia progressed. She is my rock!

African American Autoethnographic Insider–Outsider Status Considerations of Inquiry

A researcher's positional orientation is important when inquiring within and without of their culture of origin. In light of the perilous history African Americans have endured at the hand of research, it is no wonder that currently so many African Americans remain suspicious and distrustful about research participation (Scharff et al., 2010). Examining our respective and complex statuses compared to participants is particularly necessary when inquiring of African American participants, in general, and a husband caring for his wife experiencing dementia, in particular, as the inquiry pertains to autoethnography. A strategy to achieve this is insider–outsider status analysis.

While precluded from full access to insider status in understanding the realities (Collins, 1991) of Black womanhood because of social, worldview, and anatomical differences, as a husband, I have found that my wife's lived experiences have touched my life in immeasurable ways. Although I recognize this view is evolving, it is one held by this husband–wife perspective. James Banks (2006) postulates a typology of four researcher orientations: "indigenous-insider, indigenous-outsider, external-insider, and external-outsider" (pp. 179–181).

Banks's (2006) typology was introduced as a tool to assess a researcher's positionality in conducting cross-cultural research. The typology is instrumental in helping researchers discern the targeted culture and assessing their proximity to the population of inquiry. Theoretically, the closer the cultural proximity of the researcher, the closer the insider status: Indigenous-insider and external-insider. Conversely, the farther the proximity of the researcher, Indigenous-outsider and external-outsider, the more distant are cultural understandings and knowledge. Having Indigenous status implies dichotomous birth standing: We are either born into a culture or not. It is reasonable to acknowledge, however, that birth standing alone may not assure a person insider status. We can be adopted or embrace a culture over our culture of origin. In contrast, Banks theorizes outside status as researcher-oriented. Banks seems to imply that the Indigenous-outsider status researcher takes an intentional stance, a choice, to reject birth-right affiliation and seek to replace it with "an outside or oppositional culture" (2006, p. 180). The remaining orientation is external-outsider. This researcher was born outside of the targeted culture, and that culture seems odd to him. The researcher's interest and understanding of the targeted culture of inquiry are cursory, at best, and deleterious, at worst. The researcher may find aspects of the culture interesting and may mistake a tourist perspective as reality. Ethically, this researcher's interpretations of the targeted culture should be scrutinized for bias and credibility. Important in establishing credibility in autoethnography is the researcher's path to insider status that may include acquired knowledge about the phenomenon, relationship to participants, member checking, and triangulation.

These research orientations are applicable to autoethnography in varying degrees as they intersect with the dimensions of caregiving and marriage. Gender identity notwithstanding, unique dynamics of genderedness in the male caregiving space reveal unknowns that require Indigenous-insider consultation to facilitate effective care. In the care of my wife, I was, by gender, the external-insider in terms of some of the hygiene care for my wife. However, I can claim insider marriage status.

Somatic Anxieties and Help From the Indigenous-Insider

Taking a bath had always been preferred to a shower for my wife. However, she appreciated the utility of a shower when time was an issue. When time was not an issue, she would claim alone evening time to read, soak, and relax. When I or our young children would enter her bath, time would stand still until we exited the room. Although she would not say a word, the silence prompted our quick exit of her solitude. After the diagnosis, I noticed she took fewer baths and more showers. When I started giving her a bath, the most obvious thing I noticed was how it relaxed her. Eventually, however, lifting her out of the bath became a problem because of safety issues, and it became necessary to bathe her in the shower. Except for her stepping over the curb and into the shower, bathing was an easy chore, although it did not relax her as much as her coveted soaking bath did. While I knew I did not care for her as she cared for herself in the past, I felt confident. I managed to bathe her daily until one of my wife's close friends gifted my wife lotion.

I understood the message and realized that I had not been applying lotion after bathing my wife. I also realized that my wife had different lotions (including the one her friend gifted her), creams, and baby lotion in her bathroom cabinet I had not noticed. The next time my wife's friend visited, she asked if I was using the lotion she gave us, and I replied I used it but alternated it with other creams my wife had in her cabinet. Her lotion did not have a scent to it but had a rich texture to it. In the same helpful tone, she told me that my wife's skin was still a little dry and offered several solutions. She explained that the lotion she gave my wife was moisturizing and served as a base and to put the scented creams on top of if I wanted to. She first said that daily bathing might be too much for my wife's skin since she remained at home most of the time. Next, she suggested I use a baby lotion to coat my wife's skin when she stepped out of the shower. Even though this advice worked, I felt guilty for not knowing what was obvious to my wife's friend. While not giving it much thought at the time, I later recognized it as insider knowledge that I value and continue to seek.

Sometime after learning about moisturizers, when my wife's speech was waning, she would sometimes tell me that something hurt, when she needed to go to the bathroom, for example. But she touched her breast and uttered the words "It hurts . . ." Immediately, I assumed something like cancer. At this time, she was still wearing a bra. I removed her shirt and her bra to feel for what I had only heard about. I did not feel any lump, so I looked closely under her breast and saw that at the back of her breast it was red and raw. Through my panic, I applied an antibiotic cream. This seemed to relieve her pain. After I dressed her, I called and made an appointment with her doctor. I also called a female Registered Nurse (RN) relative, and she gave me options that were similar to the directions my wife's doctor gave me. But she told me the application of the antibiotic cream was fine initially but to stop applying it because the area should be dry. The doctor told me to clean and completely dry the area and then to apply a dusting of cornstarch. So, when I called my RN relative to find out where I could find cornstarch, she added to the list of options aluminum-free deodorant, baby powder, and a lotion that turned into a powder, along with several other options. I remembered using cornstarch to cook with once or twice but didn't find any in our kitchen. So, initially, I used my wife's deodorant but realized it was not aluminum-free. When I finally looked in my wife's cabinet, I found baby powder and lotion for under her breast.

As an external-insider or spouse caregiver, I felt confident in my wishes to care for my wife but had to become more competent through Indigenous-insiders' knowledge and understanding. In writing autoethnography, Banks's (2006) typology provides a distance gauge that helps researchers determine where a guide or docent who explains issues we may not have the experience to understand but, without it, makes our inquiry weak is needed. Another aspect of utilizing an insider is to give credibility to the interpretation of data. In my case, care knowledge was triangulated (Fusch et al., 2018) across sources by three insider informants in brief, impromptu queries.

Reader Thought Questions and Further Reading

1. Why was the institutional review board created? What is its role?
2. What are ethical considerations in qualitative research and autoethnography?
3. How did the author address his ethical concerns?
4. What strategies did the author use to address ethical concerns?
5. What have been the historical experiences of Black Americans in research and experimentation?
6. Compare and contrast Tullis's guiding ethical questions to the author's.
7. What are the risks and vulnerabilities in autoethnography?
8. What does the author mean by insider outsider status? What role did insider status play in caregiving for his wife?
9. What are ethical concerns in disclosure?
10. What does the author mean by "triangulation" in the chapter?

References

Anabo, I. F., Elexpuru-Albizuri, I., & Villardon-Gallego, L. (2019). Revisiting the Belmont Report's ethical principles in internet-mediated research: Perspectives from disciplinary associations in the social sciences. *Ethics and Information Technology, 21*, 137–149. https://doi.org/10.1007/s10676-018-9495-z

Andrews, S. (2017). *Searching for an autoethnographic ethic.* Routledge.

Banks, J. A. (2006). *Cultural diversity and education: Foundations, curriculum and teaching.* Pearson.

Bochner, A. P., & Ellis, C. (2016). *Evocative autoethnography: Writing lives and telling stories.* Routledge.

Chatham-Carpenter, A. (2010). "Do thyself no harm": Protecting ourselves as authoethnographers. *Journal of Research Practice, 6*(1), Article M1. http://search.ebscohost.com.pvamu.idm.oclc.org/login.aspx?direct=true&db=eric&AN=EJ902230

Collins, P. H. (1991). Learning from the outsider within: The sociological signific. In M. M. Fonow & J. A. Cook (Eds.), *Beyond methodology: Feminist scholarship as lived research* (pp. 35–59). Indiana University Press.

Dougas, K., & Carless, D. (2013). A history of autoethnographic inquiry. In Handbook of autoethnography. In S. H. Jones, T. Adams, & C. Ellis (Eds.), *Handbook of Autoethnography* (pp. 84–106). Routledge.

Dunbar, P. L. (1895). We wear the mask. In *The complete poems of Paul Laurence Dunbar* (p. 54). Dodd, Mead and Company.

Ferngren, G. (2017). Vivisection ancient and modern. *History of Medicine, 4*(3), 211–221. doi:10.17720/2409-5834.v4.3.2017.02b

Fisher, J. A. (2007). Coming Soon to a physician near you: Medical neoliberalism and pharmaceutical clinical trials. *Harvard Health Policy, 8*(1), 61–70.

Fusch, P., Fusch, G. E., & Ness, L. R. (2018). Denzin's paradigm shift: Revising triangulation in research. *Journal of Social Change, 10*, 19-32.

Gamble, V. N. (1997). Under the shadow of Tuskegee: African Americans and health care. *American Journal of Public Health, 87*(11), 1773–1778.

Grady, D. (2007, January 23). White doctors, Black subjects: Abuse disguised as research, Book Review. *The New York Times*, F5, F8.

Harris, Y., Gorelick, P. B., Samuels, P., & Bempong, I. (1996). Why African Americans may not be participating in clinical trials. *Journal of the National Medical Association, 88*(10), 630-634. Retrieved from https://www.ncbi.nlm.nih.gov/pubmed/8918067

Jonsen, A. R. (1984). Policy and human research. In J. M. Humber & R. F. Almeder (Eds.), *Biomedical ethics reviews: 1984* (pp. 3–22). Springer Science & Business Media.

Lincoln, Y. S., & Guba, E. G. (1985). *Naturalistic inquiry.* Sage.

Miles, S. H. (2005). *The Hippocratic Oath and the ethics of medicine.* Oxford University Press.

National Commission for the Protection of Human Subjects of Biomedical and Behavioral Research. (1979). *The Belmont Report: Ethical principles and guidelines for the protections of human subjects of research.* https://www.hhs.gov/ohrp/regulations-and-policy/belmont-report/index.html

Rubinstein, R. L., & Medeiros, K. D. (2014). Successful aging, gerontological theory and neoliberlism: A qualitative critique. *Gerontologist, 55*(1), 34–42. doi:10.1093/geront/gnu080

Scharff, D. P., Mathews, K. J., Jackson, P., Hoffsuemmer, J., Martin, E., & Edwards, D. (2010). More than Tuskegee: Understanding mistrust about research participation. *Journal of Health Care for the Poor and Underserved, 21*(3), 879–897. doi:10.1353/hpu.0.0323

Skloot, R. (2011). *The Immortal Life of Henrietta Lacks.* New York: Routledge.

Tamas, S. (May 17, 2019). *Autoethnographic ethics: Resources for reframing (workshop)* [Paper presentation]. International Congress of Qualitative Inquiry, University of Illinois, Champaign-Urbana.

Teall, E. K. (2014). Medicine and doctoring in ancient Mesopotania. *Grand Valley Journal of History, 3*(1), Article 2. https://scholarworks.gvsu.edu/gvjh/vol3/iss1/2/

Tullis, J. A. (2013). Self and others: Ethics in autoethnographic research. In S. H. Jones, T. E. Adams, & C. Ellis (Eds.), *Handbook of autoethnography* (pp. 244–261). Routledge.

Washington, H. A. (2006). *Medical apartheid: The dark history of medical experimentation on Black Americans from colonial times to the present.* New York: Anchor Books.

Winau, R. (1994). The hippocratic oath and ethics in medicine. *Forensic Science International, 69*(3), 285–289. doi:10.1016/0379-0738(94)90393-x

Chapter 3

From Caring to Caregiving

Consider it pure joy, my brothers and sisters,
whenever you face trials of many kinds ...

JAMES 1:2, NIV

My obsessions with hoping my wife would miraculously be her previous self bound me to thoughts that wore me out. Constantly, I looked for signs of my old wife. I saw real glimpses of her when dementia was not part of our lives. She never took naps; neither did she now. She started explaining a complicated issue but became lost in the explanation. I tried to give her hints so she could finish her thoughts, but I finished them for her. More and more, she did not recognize rooms in our house, or when we went walking outside, she did not recognize our house and asked, "Who lives here?" I told her, "We live here," and reminded her when we bought it. I went on to tell her our children's ages when we moved in. I was fascinated by her excitement when she saw old things that seemed new to her in the moment. These conversations filled our days for some time until she became nonverbal and unable to speak and could no longer walk distances. Intellectually, I knew this would not happen and that it was irrational thought. But it had become my pathos and glimpses of how she was faded every day. I knew it was a sadness I would have to work through if I wanted to feel joy. For He told me how to have His joy (John 15:11, NIV). But how could I feel joy when my wife's mind was dying but her body was alive?

As I explored everything I could about my wife's type of dementia, I sadly realized that little scientific advancement had taken place since I studied the medical phenomenon 26 years ago as a graduate student. At that time, in spite of voluminous information on dementia, no cure had been found, but I believed medical science would find a cure in the future. Except for rarely coming into contact with persons who experienced dementia in my internship, I did not really know much about the diagnosis until later when people in my family and community experienced it. The sparse exposure I had with this diagnosis that I had gained during staffing and the development of rehabilitation plans during my graduate school internship at a rehabilitation hospital. As my career progressed, and through clinical exchanges as a rehabilitation counselor, I learned through training and exposure about individuals who experienced dementia as a result of a traumatic brain injury and neurological disorders. Despite the massive amount of textbook information on dementias, two constants remained the same over time: Her cognition was not expected to improve, and there was not a cure for dementia. Much of what I experienced up to my wife's cognitive deterioration was from a distance and I had not perceived it as a personal reality. Eventually, I realized I could ensure a quality of life for us that allowed my wife to gracefully ease into the darkness of dementia. So, after considering the science of dementia, I focus on the art of caregiving.

Prevailing Knowledge at the Diagnosis of My Wife

Dementia is the reason for the central phenomenon of this book: caregiving. In a broad sense, dementia is a decline in mental ability and refers to a group of disorders impacting memory, thinking, and social behaviors that significantly alter activities of daily living (ADLs) from what is considered normal behavior. The abnormal brain changes result in a decline in cognitive capacity and interfere with independent functioning. Dementia is nonspecific and is estimated to be caused by 13 types of diseases (Heerena, 2019). These include Alzheimer's disease (AD), vascular disease, Parkinson's disease, Lewy bodies, Wernicke-Korsakoff syndrome, Creutzfeldt-Jakob disease (also called mad cow disease), frontotemporal dementia (FTD), Huntington's disease, HIV/AIDS, fatal familial insomnia, mixed dementia, chronic traumatic encephalopathy (brain injury), and normal pressure hydrocephalus. Alzheimer's dementia is the most common type, with FTD being the second most common type. I am the caregiver for my wife who experiences moderate early-onset FTD. She was formally diagnosed in 2011 at the age of 53, and her doctor and I believe it may have started in 2005 at the age of 47, with some indications it may have started before then.

FTD was first discussed in 1892 by Arnold Pick, a physician, when he described a 71-year-old patient with premature cognitive deterioration symptoms in loss of language (Pick et al., 1997). As in the aforementioned case, Pick documented subsequent cases in which significant frontal and temporal lobe degeneration of the brain was evident. By the 1920s, the term "Pick's disease" (Dickerson, 2014, p. 176) emerged as the precursor to FTD. This classification refers to a group of diseases including "behavior variant FTD" (bvFTD), "semantic dementia (SD) or the semantic variant" of the primary progressive aphasia (PPA) type. Early-onset dementia, known as frontotemporal lobar degeneration (FTLD), is typically diagnosed in individuals 45 to 65 years of age. This regional brain degeneration is the result of nerve cell damage and, as a consequence, causes impaired functioning in behavior, personality, and overall generative and receptive language functioning.

The two primary diseases that cause frontotemporal degeneration are the "protein tau," which causes a group of brain disorders, and the "TDP43" protein, which also causes a group of brain disorders. The etiology of the focus on the brain's frontal and temporal lobes are still a mystery to scientists.

The rates of dementia are growing substantially in the United States. Despite this growth, accurate information about the incidence and prevalence of dementia cannot be determined because national databases do not exist. Researchers must rely on regional studies that, in some instances, only assess one racial or ethnic group. Other limiting factors include incongruent age, assessment, and diagnostic measures data sets between studies (Mehta & Yeo, 2019). My wife's type of dementia is FTD with PPA. It appears in people 45 and 65 years of age but can appear as early as when people are in their 20s or as late as their 80s. Very rough prevalence estimates suggest 50,000 to 60,000 people experience FTD in the United States (Alzheimer's Association, 2019).

The incidence and prevalence of dementia for African Americans are reported to be more than the collective total number of all other ethnic or racial groups. On the other hand, African Americans live longer after being diagnosed with dementia, primarily AD. New African American cases in the United States, based on 14 studies reported by Mehta and Yeo (2019), are estimated to be, on average yearly, 2.6% (SD = 1%>). Although the total numbers of African American cases are not available for the United States, a Mississippi study reports dementia from <0.01% in women in the 40–50 age range to 68.1% in 100-year-old individuals (Schoenberg et al., 1985). Varying rates are reported by other regional studies that make dementia prevalence uncertain.

Dickerson (2014) criticizes that incidence and prevalence rates of FTD are understudied. Citing Knopman et al. (2004), Dickerson reports a Rochester, Minnesota study indicating rates of "2.2 per 100,000 between ages 40 and 49, 3.3 per 100,000 between ages 50 and 59, and 8.9 per 100,000 between ages 60 and 69" (p. 177). Dickerson suggests classification complexity as a reason for this lack of clarity.

In another study conducted by Plassman and colleagues (2007), the researchers sought to estimate the prevalence of AD and other dementias in the United States using a nationally representative sample. In terms of this book and its focus of exploring caregiving for my wife who experiences dementia, this study is significant in that it represents the prevailing knowledge and diagnostic practices for dementia. The Aging, Demographics, and Memory Study (ADAMS; Plassman et al., 2007) was the methodology used to sample 856 individuals for the study (see Plassman et al., 2007, for specific selection concerns, criteria, and design details). Within the selection was the assessment and diagnosis of dementia. This information was collected during a home visit and included the cognitive, functional, and medical history features; a list of medications; present neuropsychiatric symptoms; functional diminished cognition; and a history of diminished cognition in the family. Additionally, measures administered during the home visit were a neuropsychological battery (Langa et al., 2005, pp. 181–191, as reported by Plassman et al., 2007), a self-reported depression rating, a standardized neurological examination, a blood pressure measurement, collection of buccal DNA samples for apolipoprotein E (APOE) genotyping, and a video recording of the earlier-listed measures. Following the collection of the previously mentioned patient information, a meeting was convened by a geropsychiatrist, a neurologist, a neuropsychologist, a cognitive neuroscientist, nurses, and neuropsychology technicians who assigned a preliminary research diagnosis of cognitive status. A final diagnosis was provided by a consensus expert panel of neuropsychologists, neurologists, geropsychiatrists, and internists. The diagnoses were characterized into three areas: normal cognitive functioning, cognitively impaired but not demented, and dementia. A diagnosis of dementia was based on the *Diagnostic and Statistical Manual of Mental Disorder, Third Edition, Revised* (*DSM-III-R*; American Psychiatric Association, 1987) and the *DSM-IV* (American Psychiatric Association, 1994) criteria. Other diagnostic determinations were based on *DSM* criteria but included the clinical judgment of the consensus panel.

As a result of the Plassman et al. (2007) study, an estimate of 3.8 million individuals in the United States experience dementia, and more than 2.5 million experience AD. With the use of the ADAMS, Plassman and colleagues supplied the first prevalence estimate of dementia. Although the study indicated that the prevalence across studies was problematic because of the variance in the age categories reported, age was the most robust predictor of dementia in the ADAMS. Additionally, another strong prediction factor in this study was the higher an individual's education level, the lower the risk. In contrast to other studies (Bachman et al., 1992; Launer et al., 1999), women in the Plassman et al. study did not experience a greater risk of dementia than men. Similarly, while other studies (Perkins et al., 1997; Tang et al., 2001) and literature (Manly & Mayeux, 2004; Mehta & Yeo, 2019) reported a higher rate of dementia for African Americans, in the Plassman et al. study, when controlling for education, gender, and APOE genotype, the odds ratio was still elevated but not statistically significant. It is unclear if this outcome is biased. However, a concern in the interpretation of the overall data as it relates to African Americans is the statement "the lack of neuroimaging and other medical tests for all participants may have influenced the accuracy with non-AD dementias were identified" (Plassman et al., 2007, p. 130). Questions emerge as to why this information was not provided by the study to facilitate inclusion. As my wife's caregiver, I am aware that experiencing dementia is unavoidably expensive, even with insurance. In previous research led by Plassman and colleagues (2006), all the participants were intended to be Caucasian. In the 2007 Plassman study, 16 of the 23 participants were Caucasian Americans, thereby questioning, as Plassman et al. did, the generalizability of it to African Americans. A phenomenon revealed by Mehta and Yeo (2019) is that African Americans are less likely to go into a nursing home. If researchers rely on nursing homes to recruit participants, this phenomenon may be a factor for the low inclusion rates of African Americans in dementia studies. Exclusion might also be an ethical concern in light of the Belmont Report principle of justice (Friesen et al., 2017).

Diagnosis of FTD

While securing a diagnosis for my wife was relatively short, taking about 6 months, it may take considerable time. In our case, I attribute our quick diagnosis to our competent neurologist. We selected her from our medical group list. Years later, we were informed by friends that she had diagnosed their loved ones with dementia or was treating them for a different neurological condition. Except for specific neurological information, my wife's thorough, current medical history was easy to access by the neurologist. As the diagnostic process ensued, new labs included blood and urine tests called a dementia screen. I was aware of communication between my wife's primary care physician and the neurologists to rule out or identify other illnesses. Neuroimaging and other tests included a chest x-ray, magnetic resonance imaging for structural analysis, positron emission tomography, single-photon emission computed tomography, electrocardiogram, and a computerized tomography scan. As an aside, although most of these tests were covered by our insurance, they were not completely covered at the diagnostic stage. This resulted in an out-of-pocket cost of a few thousand dollars. We were blessed to be able to afford them. But I cannot help but be concerned for people who cannot afford them. My wife was seeing a psychiatrist for unexplained stomach issues that were determined to be related to anxiety and depression and were successfully treated with a low-dose antidepressant. These were a result of her dementia diagnosis and concerns and the loss of several loved ones within a short period. Delusions and hallucinations were not evident at diagnosis but surfaced postdiagnosis at the loss of our son. Our neurologist provided us with a copy of the results of my wife's neuropsychological exam. At this visit, my wife asked her if she could resume driving. At the first visit with my wife to her neurologist, she advised my wife not to drive until we received her definitive test results. So, with the results, my wife asked the question again. The neurologist stated to my wife that she should take a driving test to determine this. However, I knew that she would not be able to drive anymore. This realization made the final diagnosis even more hurtful. My wife's loss of driving independence also contributed to depression.

The diagnosis of early-onset dementia came at a crucial time in my wife's career. She was planning to return to her full-time career. She was also ABD ("all but dissertation") for her doctorate in curriculum and instruction with an emphasis on children's literature. She had been teaching English as an adjunct at the community college near our home. As a result of a reduction in workforce to close the department where she worked previously, she had been laid off from her university faculty position but asked to apply for another position. When she asked me if she should apply, we had had discussions for a few years about her yearning to be at home with our pre-teen and teen children. So she decided to step out of her career to be home with our children.

DSM-5 Diagnosis Criteria (2013). As indicated earlier, the *DSM* provides critical behavioral criteria for diagnosing frontotemporal dementia. In the fifth edition of the *DSM* (American Psychiatric Association, 2013) "neurocognitive disorders" (NCD) replaced the "dementia." This archaic nomenclature is a Latin derivative from *demens*, meaning "being out of one's mind" (Assal, 2019). Even though the term dementia remains standard jargon in the fields of psychology and psychiatry, the use of *NCD* is replacing it, thereby lessening the associated stigma. While I am aware of the usage of *NCD* in clinical and academic settings, I continue to use the term dementia when engaging with medical practitioners, colleagues, family, and friends regarding my wife's diagnosis. In addition to standard use and habit, dementia currently resonates with a clearer understanding. Furthermore, my wife's practitioners use dementia and *NCD* interchangeably in their respective clinical settings. An additional change in the *DSM-5* is the renaming of FTD to "frontotemporal lobar degeneration." This change attempts to align diagnostic criteria with emerging research terminology. Other significant changes may be accessed by reviewing the *DSM-5*.

ADLs

Experiences of my wife with dementia are aligned with the criteria in the *DSM-5* (American Psychiatric Association, 2013). Specifically, this criterion is designated below with application to my wife's experiences. While her initial diagnosis was mild under the *DSM-IV-TR* (4th ed., text revision; American Psychiatric Association, 2000) criteria, it has progressed and is now a major neurocognitive disorder. Its cumulative effect has rendered her incapable of carrying out ADLs over time. Her degenerative cognitive ability is also manifest in digressive abilities as illustrated in Table 3.1. Table 3.1 was adapted from *Activities & Instrumental Activities of Daily Living—Definitions, Importance and Assessments* (Paying for Senior Care, 2019).

The timeline in the table represents my wife's noticeable decline in ADLs. A person without cognitive or physical impairments is able to carry out basic and instrumental ADLs (IADLs; Edemekong et al., 2020). Basic ADLs include ambulating, feeding, dressing, personal hygiene, continence, and toileting. More complex thinking and organizational skills of IADLs include transportation and shopping, managing finances, shopping and meal preparation, house cleaning and home maintenance, managing communication with others, and managing medications. Consistent with ADL literature (Cahn-Weiner et al., 2002), early in her diagnosis, my wife carried out basic ADLs while her IADL skills waned.

At the top of Table 3.1, the levels of assistance are indicated. At the bottom, time periods indicate major diagnostic and major life events. The first year, 2005, indicates the year we believe my wife began experiencing decision-making difficulties but was able to function across all areas of ADLs independently. The formal diagnosis was made in 2011. In 2013, my wife's father passed. (Her mother passed in 2004.) In 2014, our son took his life. At the loss of our son, not only was a cognitive and physical decline noticeable in my wife but also an emotional decline (not represented in the table), which emerged in the form of psychosis. This is discussed in another chapter. The year 2016 marks the passing of my wife's sister, her last immediate family member. Almost total dependence for ADLs is indicated in 2020, at the writing of this book. "No noticeable decline" is coded "N." In spite of this coding, cognitive decline (in 2005) is believed to have begun occurring but was not noticeable. An example of this type of decline occurred when my wife asked me to help her manage her father's affairs as he began experiencing cognitive decline in his late 80s. The "X" code indicates a noticeable decline as the condition progressed to total dependence. The "A" code indicates a level of ability while noticeable decline was occurring.

As my wife's cognitive ability diminished over time, she became more and more indifferent and lethargic about what was occurring around us. Her affect became naturally flat; she rarely smiled. She was no longer capable of showing sympathy or empathy. Soon after my wife was diagnosed, I took her to an endocrinology exam and was informed that her lab work revealed signs of starvation. While this was a shock to me, I had not paid close attention to her eating habits before the diagnosis. I did recall that she was not eating much and attributed this behavior to

Table 3.1. *Progression of My Wife's Dementia*

ADL ↓ Assistance→	No Assistance		Some Assistance		Complete Assistance		Unable to Do
Bathing	N	N	X	A	A	X	X
Dressing	N	N	X	A	X	X	X
Grooming	N	N	X	A	X	X	X
Oral Care	N	N	X	X	X	X	X
Toileting	N	N	N	X	X	X	X
Transferring	N	N	N	X	X	X	X
Walking	N	N	N	A	A	A	X
Climbing Stairs	N	N	N	A	A	A	X
Eating	N	N	N	A	A	A	A
Shopping	N	X	X	X	X	X	X
Cooking	N	X	X	X	X	X	X
Manage Medications	N	X	X	X	X	X	X
Use Phone	N	X	X	X	X	X	X
Housework	N	X	X	X	X	X	X
Laundry	N	X	X	X	X	X	X
Driving	N	X	X	X	X	X	X
Managing Finances	N	X	X	X	X	X	X
YEAR	2005	2011	2013	2014	2016	2018	2020

Source: Adapted from *Activities & Instrumental Activities of Daily Living—Definitions, Importance and Assessment*, by Paying for Senior Care, July 11, 2019, https://www.payingforseniorcare.com/activities-of-daily-living.
Note: N = no noticeable decline; X = noticeable decline; A = declining ability.

weight maintenance. While I did not observe at diagnosis hyperorality, it has evolved to my wife putting odd things (paper clips, screws, etc.) in her mouth and hair. My daughter and I try to remove any objects near my wife.

My wife had always been an excellent communicator. So when she began to experience difficulty with the selection of words in her speech, it was noticeable, although not to a great degree. Prior to her diagnosis, it was just odd. After her diagnosis, her overall language ability was only slightly diminished and in a greater cognitive context. We believe my wife was diagnosed during the late early stage (Giebel et al., 2015) of dementia. To some extent, her articulations gave an indication of the progression of dementia. For example, as we took our common driving routes to different destinations, she might exclaim, "Were those trees always there?" Prior to the diagnosis, I might have just asked, "Yes, you don't remember them?" Or, as she walked into a room when she was experiencing moderate dementia, she would say, "This is so pretty." And the rooms in our house are pretty because she decorated them in warm and soothing colors and hues. But, every time she entered the room, it was anew. When she stopped asking these types of questions, it was because she had become nonverbal in the advanced stage of dementia.

The advanced stage of dementia has incapacitated all aspects of my wife's independence as indicated in Table 3.1. Her memory lasts for only a minute if not less. Although she might respond to a question because of intonation, she usually does not seem to understand what she is being asked. She experiences great confusion about relieving her bladder to the extent that she begins to sweat profusely and/or begins to squirm. Often, this occurs in the mid- to late afternoon and coincides with what has been characterized by her doctor as "sundowning" (Bachman & Rabins, 2006). She recognizes few people and responds to the voices of our daughter and me. I also believe my wife recognizes the spirits of our daughter and me. Nurses and other practitioners have told me that my wife becomes more alert and responsive when we come into a room or when we ask her to do things. I have worked on talking to my wife in a quiet, soothing voice. Additionally, I believe part of this is because my wife's visual perception and acuity have diminished significantly. For example, this is seen in impaired depth perception when climbing and descending stairs of the same color and in seeing food on her plate. She no longer recognizes objects in our house. She is uninterested in her pastime of watching television and can no longer follow what is on it. We try not to make quick movements because she is easily startled and jumps if touched unexpectedly. Although not as noticeable in the advanced stage of dementia, when we would say our prayers and I mentioned our late son's name, she would close her eyes tightly, take a deep breath, and sigh before we finished. Earlier, she would ask, "Who is that?" When I would tell her that he was our son who died, she would ask during the early stage, "How did he die?" When I would tell her, "He took his life." She would try to ask a follow-up question but could not finish the question because she did not appear to remember what she was asking.

Her ability to walk has been severely impaired during the advanced stage to the point of requiring a wheelchair to move around our house.

She is dependent on our daughter, attendant, or me for all transfers. My daughter and I bathe her daily or every other day. She experiences muscle rigidity in her upper extremities and postural instability.

Journey From Caring to Caregiving

> *But they that wait upon the* LORD *shall renew their strength; they shall mount up with wings as eagles; they shall run, and not be weary; and they shall walk, and not faint.*
>
> ISAIAH 40:31, KJV

> *But he said to me, "My grace is sufficient for you, for my power is made perfect in weakness." Therefore I will boast all the more gladly of my weaknesses, so that the power of Christ may rest upon me.*
>
> II CORINTHIANS 12:9

In 2011, my wife was diagnosed with early-onset FTD by a neurologist after brain scans and neuropsychological testing. Even though the brain scans showed no evidence of the disorder, neurological testing revealed marked impaired functioning. After discussing my wife's behavior, the neurologist and I determined that the disorder probably could be traced back to at least 2005 and even earlier. But the neurologist did not know the etiology of the condition. She offered that FTD is believed to result from a loss of protein in the brain, as stated previously. I believe she tried to break it down into layperson's language for me and I appreciated that.

Caring for Each Other

Dementia and Relationships

Prior to graduate school, I nebulously understood dementia to be a neurological disorder that impacted people later in their lives. I understood it was not an eminent end point for everyone, but in most cases, cognitive decline could not be reversed. Before then, around my high school years, my understanding of dementia formed in silhouette as I came into contact with people exhibiting what was loosely defined as deviant behavior. I remember infrequently hearing people use the term *demented* to describe an adult's behavior as bizarre in a pejorative way and possibly connoting evil behavior. Recalling the target of the slang, I remember the person being described this way as being adrift. He was in society but not socially fitting into society in a functional way. I remember an elderly family member who stayed away from everyone in a different room and would only come into the room when called. I noticed the spouse would, in a conversational tone, direct the person to do different things. Although I did not understand his behavior, I saw this person giving care to his spouse. Because of my youth, the relationship seemed one-sided, with one person telling the other person what to do. It seemed odd and cold to me. The person being cared for died a week after their caregiver-spouse's death.

Another person with obvious cognitive impairment and inside my broader family circle was managed and protected by multiple family members in a rural setting. This person had a quiet manner; was always well groomed, fed, and sheltered; and appeared normal until the person's strange behavior emerged. Even though this person was included in activities and sat in the gathering space, this person interacted with family and friends on the peripheral. Growing up, we were always told to say hello to this person, and we did. And the person said hello back, as directed. From an early age, when we entered his space, we were told to sit and talk with this person. The person seemed to talk to someone not present. I noticed that when I asked a question, the person recognized the interrogative nature of the question and might laugh, but the response was nonsensical and gibberish, with some discernable words but little to no syntactical meaning. I also recognized the person would respond to a yes–no question with "yes" or "no," and during my youth, I believed the person was trying to engage in the conversation at hand. As I spent more time with him and over time, usually at a family gathering, I saw the person answer the television with a "yes" and a quick laugh. I recognized the person only perceived enough of the dialogue to form some type of semantic response, although crude. But if the person engaged in unsafe behavior like leaving the space, a family member would appear from nowhere and redirect the person in such a way as to not draw attention to the person. When I eventually asked what happened to the person, I was given a definitive experience and period of time that marked when his behavior began to change. The origin of the behavior was believed to have a start date after a traumatic experience. I looked forward to seeing him, if only to sit quietly.

It was not until my master's degree program that I began to formally learn about dementia. In my graduate studies in rehabilitation counseling, dementia was briefly addressed as a degenerative neurological disorder. More focus was placed on AD than other dementias. Today, the second-most common dementia to Alzheimer's is frontotemporal lobular degeneration.

Remembering Back While Moving Forward

One of the earliest indications of my wife's cognitive decline was evident in her watching and following events on our television. My wife loved watching TV and almost anything cinematic. In fact, one of our earliest joint purchases after we were married (June 1983) was a 19-inch color television. This replaced my 9-inch black-and-white TV. By around 1998 and a few TVs later, for my birthday, I asked for a 36-inch console TV, and my wife was happy to oblige. I really wanted a larger screen, but we made a decision based on cost and placement in the room. The technology was a factor too, as it had not progressed to the point of a clear picture from anywhere in the room. At that time, picture clarity could only be achieved from about three angles in the room, with the best view directly in front of the television.

As I think back to around 2005, I realize that my wife began to rewind shows on our 36-inch console TV. Initially, this was not noticeable because she would walk out of the room, walk back in, rewind, and state she wanted to see what she missed. At first, this happened seemingly infrequently as she attended to our children or she purposefully went from room to room in our house to put something up or clean. Eventually, when she sat in the living room, she would ask about the action on the show and I would attempt to explain it to her. This behavior became more and more frequent. Over time and barely noticeable, and while sitting for periods, she began to ask every few minutes, "What did he/she say?" or "What just happened?" Not connecting this to cognitive decline, I would become irritated and would quip to her, "Pay attention." Also, rather than rewinding the TV herself, she asked me to rewind. I now attribute the rewinding to behavior consistent with the progression of dementia. And I saw this request to be odd, as she had always been independent. This might have marked my wife's recognition that something was wrong, although imperceptible to both of us, and her reaching out to me to become her caregiver (Valois &

Galvin, 2014), even if in the moment it was just to assist her with the TV remote, represented a discernible pattern. Other subtle indications that she was asking me to provide caregiving included her asking me for a recipe for dishes she had made countless times. Because she and I shared cooking and other household chores, her lapse in memory went unnoticed. Looking back, when we were in the kitchen together and she asked me to prepare a dish she had made many times, this might have been another example of her subconsciously seeking help for her cognitive struggles. Although in hindsight this makes sense, it was just odd at the time.

Emerging Communication Issues

Once diagnosed and as my wife's condition progressed, caregiving became a major part of my life. As my wife's independence was coming to an end, my daughter and I struggled with doing too much for her and tried to find a balance so she can maintain her autonomy. We, nonetheless, observed her growing frustrations when we would try to help her dress; she would resist by saying she could do it. I soon recognized that some of her resistance had to do with my approach to dressing her. For example, rather than asking her to raise her arm to put into a top, I began lifting her arm to put it into her top. The resistance was twofold: On one hand, the absence of a verbal prompt to her to allow me to help her put on her clothes did not prepare her for what was about to happen, and this did not make sense to her. And even when she understood the nonverbal prompt, she struggled to cooperate because the task seemed nonsensical because she felt she could do this by herself. But when I say to my wife, "Let's lift your arm," she is 100% more cooperative in achieving the task. Speaking softly and slowly also made a huge difference. When I assumed the role of my wife's primary caregiver, particularly as her dementia progressed, analyzing every task to achieve an action was a big challenge but became easier over time. As she became less and less able to predict how she could assist in her care and more dependent on me to accomplish all her ADLs.

Caregiving

Caregiving is sometimes confused with *caretaking*. The two terms are differentiated as the former meaning receiving love, care, and affection, while the latter relates to an object receiving attention for the purpose of maintenance. The recipient of caregiving is a loved one and someone in need of being looked after (Valois & Galvin, 2014). In contrast, the object of caretaking is an inanimate object such as property, a house, a yard or garden, or even a cemetery. With either, the person providing the care engages in a labor of love. In caregiving to a loved one, the labor is performed for a child or a person who requires help meeting individual needs or ADLs as listed in Table 3.1. Caregivers provide a range of services that may fall on a continuum from nonessential assistance to essential life-or-death services. For example, all caregiving for my infant son was essential. Nonessential caregiving might include cooking a meal for my teenage son or driving him to a basketball game. In contrast, providing caregiving to my wife who experiences dementia is essential as she experiences early, mild to moderate, and severe/advanced levels (Giebel et al., 2015).

In viewing caregiving from a critical perspective, as my wife's dementia has progressed to her becoming less independent and verbal, it has become increasingly apparent to me that my way of providing caregiving requires intentionality for axiological or moral reasons. Specifically, I have found it necessary to remind myself to be intentionally verbal when I am in her space. When caring for my wife it becomes easy to go through the motions of caregiving (see Table 3.2) and ignore her as a person. Positioning her as an object (Rocco, 2005) to only be dressed, bathed, groomed, fed, medicated, and moved from location to location has been a challenge. While my caregiving behaviors are important and life-sustaining, alone they ignore my wife's personhood and our relationship. The field of nursing provides the relational practice of embodiment (Fernandez, 2020) rather than objectification when providing care.

Caregivers may be unpaid or paid; family members, friends, companions, or strangers; or a combination of these. Valois and Galvin (2014) differentiate levels of caregiving as "formal and informal" (p. 610). Basically, the difference is paid and unpaid. Formal caregivers are "paid" and typically are considered trained professionals and may be strangers to the recipient of care. This type of caregiver may be hired through an agency or be an independent contractor. Informal caregivers are "unpaid" and tend to be family and close friends. Although much of my wife's care is provided by me, my daughter provides care for a significant amount of time. Two paid caregivers have provided care for my wife over time.

Neither were strangers. Both worked full-time in professional caregiving careers. One of the caregivers had cleaned our house for years before assuming the role of caregiver. She and my wife were friends and would spend time together shopping and doing other things. We knew that in addition to her full-time job at a local hospital, she also worked part-time as a caregiver. While both caregivers were trained, our friend was instrumental in advising us on many issues that ensured my wife's quality of life. Regrettably, she passed away from cancer.

The level of caregiving for my wife has changed and depends on her needs and the capacity of the caregiver. Critical to providing formal caregiving for my wife is the attribute of moral capaciousness that embodies a sense of duty to meet my wife's needs. Understanding this capacity in my role as primary and informal caregiver has evolved as my wife's dementia has progressed. Additionally, my arranging caregiving has changed from at the diagnosis, leaving my wife at home unattended to some monitoring by my son, my daughter, and myself to around-the-clock care. Paramount to caregiving for my wife was not only providing vital attention but also ensuring a quality of life. It pains me whenever I perceive her to be in the slightest discomfort. I feel intense hurt when she is in any pain because she cannot communicate to me or I cannot figure it out. Of course, the guilt of not achieving a high quality of care may be irrational thought, but it's how I feel. This high standard creates mental and maybe even emotional dissonance because I have chosen to continue to work. Consequently, I have to rely on others to provide care for my wife when I have to be away from home. Our son provided significant attention to his mother before he passed. Until then, when he was not in school or working, he mainly made sure his mother ate on time, accompanied her on short walks, took her to minor appointments, ran errands for her, and the like. As a result of his passing, my wife's dementia turned psychotic quickly, and she began to require constant care and monitoring because of the emergence of wandering behavior. Even though I had worked with people who were psychotic, my feeling of helplessness broke my heart.

So after prayer and careful selection, I have realized that I need to trust others to care for her. The other caregivers include our daughter and attendants we've hired to attend to her needs. One factor that helps relieve my stress is our security monitoring system. Before our son passed, our home alarm system was not monitored. When wandering behavior became an issue with my wife, we upgraded our home security system by installing cameras throughout our house and around our property. Now our alarm panels alert us to the opening of any door that leads to the outside and all windows. Fortunately, she has not tried to climb out of any windows. I find solace in being able to monitor my wife from different rooms in the house, even though someone is with my wife all of the time. Even though being in the room with her calms her and I try not to be away from her for more than 15 to 20 minutes, the cameras allow me to observe her in our upstairs bedroom while I am downstairs in the kitchen preparing her meal or in other rooms cleaning, washing clothes, or completing other chores.

My Typical Caregiving Schedule

My caregiving daily schedule is meant to occur with or without my participation. Table 3.2 represents a schedule that occurred around the time of the writing of this book. In reality, it is much messier than it appears. While all the items are important, the schedule is more of a checklist. It has changed as my wife's dementia has progressed. Previously, her day might have begun between 7 and 8 a.m. The schedule in Table 3.2 constantly adjusts based on when my wife wakes in the morning and when she falls asleep. On the day of Table 3.2, she woke up at 2 p.m. Unless we have a doctor's appointment or another engagement, we allow her to sleep until she wakes up. Also, she lies awake and still in the bed during the night. When she wakes me up between 4 and 5 a.m. to take her to the bathroom, I stay up to do some university work, clean, and tidy the house. Additionally, cleaning occurs throughout the day. When I started planning my wife's meals, I relied on frozen food for each meal because of convenience. After my wife's annual physical revealed that she was prediabetic, with a sodium level at the top of the acceptable range, I knew I needed to change her diet. After talking with someone in our personal support[1] system, I decided to prepare her meals ahead of time for 3 to 5 days. As a result of this important change, she is no longer in the diabetic range and her A1c decreased below the prediabetic range. Because she is no longer able to maneuver a spoon to eat oatmeal and yogurt, we feed her breakfast. As the dementia

---

1 Personal support system: composed of family and friends who have experience and/or medical training such as physicians, nurses, nursing aides.

has progressed, her visual perception has diminished significantly and interferes with her ability to see her food. Increasingly, after she attempts to eat her meals, and to alleviate frustration, I, our daughter, or an attendant will feed her the remainder. More and more frequently, she is not able to pick up her food with a knife or spoon. When she is served foods like mashed potatoes, macaroni and cheese, and rice, we feed them to her with a spoon. As often as possible, we serve my wife finger foods like chicken breast, cut into bite-sized pieces.

Table 3.2. *Caregiving Selected Daily Schedule in Advanced/Severe Dementia*

Time	Activity
4–5 a.m.	Bathroom,[1] 1st AM Med,[2] Work, Cleaning, Monitor
6–8 a.m.	Bathroom, 2nd AM Med, Work, Cleaning, Monitor
8–9 a.m.	Work, Cleaning, Housework, Laundry, Food Prep—Breakfast[3]
9–11 a.m.	Laundry, Food Prep—Lunch/Dinner,[4] Bathroom
12–2 p.m.	Laundry, Water, Bathroom
2–4 p.m.	Water, Bathroom, Feed Breakfast, Bath and Wash and Comb Hair
4–5 p.m.	Lunch, Bathroom
6–7 p.m.	Water, Bathroom
8–9 p.m.	Dinner Snack,[5] Evening, Medication, Bathroom
9–10 p.m.	In Bed, Bathroom
10–12 a.m.	In Bed, Bathroom

[1] All bathroom transfers are from the bed/recliner to wheelchair to go to bathroom; transfers in bathroom are back to the bed/recliner.

[2] First and second medications are given with 4 ounces of apple juice and 4 ounces of water. Neither can be taken with food.

[3] Breakfast: Quaker Oats with a pinch of pink sea salt, a dash of cinnamon, two raspberries, ¼ cup of blueberries, and 8 ounces of diet cranberry juice.

[4] Lunch: Sam's rotisserie chicken, one small roasted potato, mixed vegetables—three individual plates—and 8 ounces of vitamin and electrolyte water.

[5] Dinner Snack: cheese, apple, crackers, sliced turkey, yogurt, 8 ounces of water.

FROM CARING TO CAREGIVING

Responding to the Unexpected

Electrolytes, sodium, and glucose have been tricky from a chemical and nutritional level. As my wife has become more and more nonverbal to the point of very limited communication about her well-being and how she feels, we have had to learn how to care for her through trial and error. We have restricted dietary substances such as sugar and salt to avoid diabetes and high blood pressure. Well, I managed them too well. At different times, usually in the morning when my wife wakes up, she seems too listless in an unnatural way. The first time that my wife experienced this, I was out of town and our daughter was caring for her while I was away. When our daughter frantically called me, we talked, and eventually, we decided to take her blood pressure and discovered the top number to be very low. I, in turn, frantically contacted a medical professional in our personal support system, told her what was happening, and asked her to contact our daughter. When I contacted my daughter, she told me that our friend told her to give her mother sea salt. When I called about an hour later, my daughter informed me that my wife's blood pressure was rising, and eventually it reached the normal range. A few months before this incident, we had a scare when my wife collapsed outside after going to the beauty shop and had to be transported by ambulance to the emergency room. She was quickly diagnosed with a dangerously low potassium level. A friend experienced a similar event with her spouse. As a result of this experience, with her first meal, we add a pinch of sea salt and monitor her salt intake so that she gets the daily recommendation of this mineral.

A few months after the sea salt experience, my wife was once again lethargic when I got her out of bed. I took her blood pressure, and it was in the normal range. I took her temperature, and it was in the normal range. After ruminating on the possible cause, and right before I called our friend from our support system and my wife's general practitioner, I saw my bag with a diabetes blood glucose meter inside. When I retracted the needle and poked my wife, she retracted her hand but not before I got enough for a sample reading. Her glucose level was 53. Because I am a diet-controlled diabetic, I knew this was very low. I explained the reading to my daughter, and I asked her to get some apple juice from the kitchen downstairs. After my wife drank the apple juice, her glucose level rose to the normal range. From that day on, I give my wife apple juice with her first medications and either another apple juice or a sugar-free drink to take with her second medications. Although her glucose level occasionally drops, giving her apple juice seems to maintain her glucose in the normal range.

As Table 3.2 indicates, water and liquid intake are crucial. However, I have noticed that water alone does not replenish or keep electrolytes at an acceptable level. This became apparent when my wife had her first visit to the emergency room after collapsing outside of the beauty shop where she got her hair done. At the hospital, we were told that her electrolytes, in addition to her potassium, were low. After this, we added drinks with electrolytes to her water diet. Although modest, these drinks seem to help her appear more alert. Early after my wife's language began to decline, we began giving her about 16 ounces of liquid that has vitamins and electrolytes in it daily. Throughout the rest of the day, we give my wife water. We did this because she began to experience unexplainable and profuse sweating. We talked to her doctor, who could not discern the origin of the sweats but ruled out menopause. We knew that sometimes the sweats signaled that she needs to go to the bathroom, but sweats did not always signal this need. One thing we observed was that the sweats drained her. It was around this time that we added more drinks with enhanced vitamins and electrolytes. Anytime she drank a liquid or ate, we took her to the bathroom. As Table 3.2 indicates, all of her bathroom visits are labor-intensive because she has to be lifted and placed several times.

Financial Cost of Caregiving

The cost of caregiving is a persistent issue and cannot be ignored. Valois and Galvin (2014) estimate the unpaid (family and friends) cost of caregiving in the home to be $375 billion a year. They estimate that this amount is close to the doubled combined cost of home care and nursing home services at $158 billion a year. Specifically, caregiving for individuals who experience dementia is estimated at $172 billion a year.

Outside of caregiving, deductibles for office and home dental and medical visits, home health care, and medication present sizable expenses. Durable care supplies that include incontinence underwear, bed and furniture padding, and others are purchased on a regular basis.

To accommodate my wife's accessibility needs, we incorporated a "universal design" (Hamrale, 2016) to open up home spaces to accommodate my wife's ease of movement. I was aware of this type of design and had observed its utility in public and commercial spaces. I had limited knowledge of universal design in homes and relied on architect friends to inform me of this type of design. As our home was built with an open concept, much of our renovation did not require moving or removing walls. We widened door entrances to bathrooms to accommodate her wheelchair. One area of concentration was the renovation of our bedroom en suite bathroom. Initially, it was compartmentalized with a toilet room. Diagonally across the room was the curbed shower area with a door and wall separating it from the sinks, vanities, tub, and other parts of the room. Our bathroom renovation included completely opening up the room by removing any walls and doors. We doubled our shower space to eventually accommodate the full rotation of a wheelchair. Along with a walk-in curb-less shower, we installed a separate walk-in tub. My wife and I talked about our bathroom renovation having a beach theme. So our floor was the color of sand, and the walls had various blue treatments to reflect the ocean and sky.

Care for the Caregiver

Years ago, I attended a workshop focusing on care for the caregiver. Although before this season I had not lived a life where I experienced exhaustion or burnout, I was familiar with the basic concept of personal care. A concept I was exposed to regarding individuals with physical disabilities, was energy conservation and maintenance. For example, a 60-year-old individual recovering from a heart attack expends significant energy while getting dressed, and this energy expenditure may prevent him from engaging in another activity for a time. So the individual would be encouraged to plan activities so that energy could be conserved and thereby available for other activities. Initially, I learned about personal energy conservation when earning my master's degree in rehabilitation counseling and was young, physically strong, and healthy with strong coping skills. Although I engaged in physical workout activities, I did not exert myself to the point of needing to rest to restore energy. The biggest challenge I had experienced until that time was the loss of my father, with my mother and other family members providing emotional support for my bereavement. This concept explains that when energy is used in one area, it is depleted and not available in other areas for a time, and it may only be available in staggered amounts until it is completely replenished. The concept of the workshop was similar and focused on physical energy conservation, except it also stressed emotional energy conservation. The workshop stressed that when we expend all or a considerable about of emotional energy caring for clients, students, and co-workers, we may not have energy for our children or our spouse. Although I was older and married with children at the time of the workshop, I still had not needed to practice the energy conservation method. I was pretty good at leaving work at work and separating my focused attention on my family when I was with them. Energy conservation is an essential consideration for my daughter and myself in our self-care when providing family care to my wife. Caregiving for my wife keeps me in perpetual motion, from providing direct care to her to cleaning, cooking, and arranging appointments. It's a good motion but exhausting. And by the time my wife gets into bed, all I want to do is sit down and close my eyes for 15 minutes. My mother, when she could, took 15 minutes during the day to rejuvenate herself. When I remembered this, it was like medicine and always gave me the second wind I needed. If I could get the 15 minutes by midday or early evening, I would be good for the rest of the day.

But on some days, getting those 15 minutes might not happen, but I would keep trying or yearning for them. With my wife in bed, I bemoaned saying our nighttime prayers. I was tired. Moving through compulsion, recalling my dad on his knees mumbling his prayers before bed. He told us to pray even if we're tired. I start the prayer my wife taught our children, "Now I lay me down to sleep. . . ." I chose this prayer because I believed my wife could participate by saying it with me. And for a long time, she did. I was surprised when, at the mention of our deceased son's name—"God bless Cody, who we'll see in heaven someday"—my wife asked, first, where he was, then who he was, and then repeated his name. She asked me two or three times how he died, and at first, I avoided giving her an answer, not knowing how she might respond. But she kept asking as though she would keep asking until she got an answer. Finally, I told her he took his life, and she said, "Oh." Sometime afterward and as the dementia progressed, she stopped asking about his death. In our prayer, she replaced saying his name with a reaction to his name. She closes her eyes tightly when I mention his name. Nevertheless, I felt compelled to say it and felt a burst of energy afterward. Before my wife's diagnosis, we said our nightly prayers separately before falling asleep in bed and, for me, not every night. After my wife's diagnosis, I decided to lead her in prayer at mealtimes and when she gets into bed. Coupled with the output of physical energy is the emotional expenditure. In this case, planning to expend physical and emotional energy is crucial to personal care. Planning includes the scheduling of respite care along with balancing activities throughout the day.

Other Caregiving Issues

The caregiving issues addressed above reflect a snapshot of the multitude of activities engaged in daily to care for my wife. Routines are nice but may be different from day to day. As indicated earlier, my wife wakes at different times. A late rising usually means that activities like meals, bathing, and water intake and her glucose levels are altered. Medication is a factor in routines. When a medication changes, my wife's wake time or the time she goes to bed is altered. Administering medication is an important activity as my wife now requires that all her pills be crushed and consumed in soft, solid food, such as yogurt, applesauce, or the like, so that they are digested. Additionally, significant issues related to the bathroom are frequent constipation, a source of which is my wife's medications, and preparing for and attending to incontinence.

As issues arise, they can be planned for and incorporated into the daily routine. For example, measures to address incontinence include multiple levels of protective layers of disposable pads on the bed, chairs, and any other sitting areas. I learned about this through a combination of education on dementia-related blogs, support groups, websites, and product reviews. For the most part, friends and family do not have experience with dementia and its related incontinence issues, so the shared experiences of strangers have been helpful. I learned about the strategy of layering for incontinence a result of reading product reviews on internet store sites. For example, I am able to make my wife's side of our split mattress differently than my side of the bed. To make her side from the beginning, I place a fitted washable waterproof mattress protector on the bed. Next, on the mattress protector, I place a washable full-length waterproof mattress topper. Next, and for comfort, I place a quilted mattress pad on top of the topper. On top of this, I place a disposable mattress pad and then a fitted sheet. On top of the fitted sheet, I place a large mattress pad topped with a disposable mattress pad. Next are the top sheet, mattress blankets, and covers. The washable pads, then, do not have to be washed daily because they have not been soiled, as I had done for some time before discovering the layering technique. While rare, if the bedding becomes soiled as a result of incontinence, then all the bedding would be replaced. The idea with the multiple layers is to be able to remove the top disposable layer when it is soiled and to easily replace it on a daily basis. For sitting areas, although only two layers are utilized, the top layer is also disposable. This technique has been beneficial in terms of protecting recliners, bedding, and chairs. It is also something that can be easy for other caregivers to manage. The disposable layers are time-saving in that, in most cases, the top disposable layer is the only one that requires daily changing, and this reduces the amount of time needed to change and wash bedding. While my wife insisted on changing all the sheets weekly, I tend to change them biweekly. I have found information from strangers who have similar experiences with dementia to be very helpful.

Kinetic Reflections

Perpetual motion was not new to me, but it was in terms of caring for my wife. It wasn't until we had our second child that my wife and I laughed about the amount of energy it took to care for two children. We agreed that our caring for one child was a breeze. In the way parents laugh at things they learned but their adult children don't yet know, my wife's father chuckled and said to us to sleep as much as possible before our first child's birth because it would be a commodity we would yearn after her birth. When reality hit us, that understanding came rushing in. It was not just sleep, however. It was the constant movement it took to care for our two children that intrigued me. On one of our bustling days, around a year after our second child, our son, was born, I commented to my wife that I didn't know where all our energy came from. It was a rhetorical comment that she took as a question. In a nerdy way, she told me I should have listened in high school physics about Newton's laws of motion. Seeing the confusion on my face, to a fault, she proceeded to recite the laws. If that was not enough, she then went on to remind me of our teacher's demonstration using Newton's Cradle, citing Newton's second law. As I turned to walk away, she lightheartedly spouted that motion creates energy and that when we move our bodies, we create (sustainable) energy, which I told her I knew. And I did, except I had not attributed it to Newton. That Christmas holiday, my wife gifted me a silver Newton's Cradle engraved with "Your Energy Source." Even though I now move from task to task throughout the day in caring for my wife without giving the motion much thought, I reflect on that even though I feel tired, taking that first step gives me physical energy. Just as my wife and I said to each other when one of us had to get up to take care of our children, I now say to myself the word *kinetic* to remind me to move for energy.

Reader Thought Questions and Further Reading

1. What is dementia, and how is it diagnosed?
2. How is dementia different from Alzheimer's disease?
3. Explain the incidence and prevalence rates for dementias in the United States. What makes these difficult to ascertain?
4. At what age might a person be diagnosed with dementia?
5. Explain the relationship between dementia and activities of daily living.
6. What changes are evident to you about how dementia changes the lives of the person affected and the family?
7. Define *caregiving*.
8. What makes caregiving a phenomenon?
9. What is significant about the typical caregiving schedule in Table 3.2?
10. Explain the difference between direct and indirect caregiving.
11. What are the financial implications for caregiving?
12. Why is self-care for the caregiver important?
13. If you know someone with a dementia, how are their experiences different from those described in this chapter?
14. What might be the risks for a person experiencing dementia without a caregiver?
15. What does the author mean by "perpetual motion?"

References

Alzheimer's Association. (2019). *Frontotemporal dementia*. https://www.alz.org/alzheimers-dementia/what-is-dementia/types-of-dementia/frontotemporal-dementia

American Psychiatric Association. (1987). *Diagnostic and statistical manual of mental disorders—revised* (3rd ed.).

American Psychiatric Association. (1994). *Diagnostic and statistical manual of mental disorders* (4th ed.).

American Psychiatric Association. (2000). *Diagnostic and statistical manual of mental disorders* (4th ed., text revision).

American Psychiatric Association. (2013). *Diagnostic and statistical manual of mental disorders* (5th ed.).

Assal, F. (2019). History of dementia. In J. Bogousslavsky, F. Bolle, & M. Iwata (Eds.), *A history of neuropsychology* (Vol. 44, pp. 118–126). Basel Karger.

Bachman, D., & Rabins, P. (2006). "Sundowning" and other temporally associated agitation states in dementia patients. *Annual Review of Medicine, 57*, 499–511. doi:10.1146/annurev.med.57.071604.141451

Bachman, D. L., Wolf, P. A., Linn, R., Knoefel, J. E., Cobb, J., Belanger, A., D'Agostino, R. B., & White, L. R. (1992). Prevalence of dementia and probable senile dementia of the Alzheimer type in the Framingham Study. *Neurology, 42*(1), 115–119. doi:10.1212/wnl.42.1.115

Cahn-Weiner, D. A., Boyle, P. A., & Malloy, P. F. (2002). Tests of executive function predict instrumental activities of daily living in community-dwelling older individuals. *Applied Neuropsychology, 9*(3), 187–191. doi:10.1207/S15324826AN0903_8

Dickerson, B. (2014). Frontotemporal dementia. In *Dementia: Comprehensive principles and practices* (pp. 176–197). Oxford University Press.

Edemekong, P. F., Bomgaars, D. L., Sukumaran, S., & Levy, S. B. (2020, June 26). Activities of daily living. In *StatPearls*. Treasure Island. https://www.statpearls.com/articlelibrary/viewarticle/17137/

Fernandez, A. V. (2020). Embodiment and objectification in illness and health care: Taking phenomenology from theory to practice. *Journal of Clinical Nursing, 29*, 4403–4412. doi:10.1111/jocn.15431

Friesen, P., Kearns, L., Redman, B., & Caplan, A. L. (2017). Rethinking the Belmont Report? *American Journal of Bioethics, 17*(7), 15–21. doi:10.1080/15265161.2017.1329482

Giebel, C. M., Sutcliffe, C., & Challis, D. (2015). Activities of daily living and quality of life across different stages of dementia: A UK study. *Aging & Mental Health, 19*(1), 63–71. doi:10.1080/13607863.2014.915920

Hamrale, A. (2016). Universal design and the problem of "post-disability" ideology. *Design and Culture, 8*(3), 285–309.

Heerena, E. (2020, January 15). *13 kinds of diseases that cause dementia symptoms and prognosis.* Very Well Health. https://www.verywellhealth.com/types-of-dementia-98770

Knopman, D. S., Petersen, R. C., Edland, S. D., Cha, R. H., & Rocca, W. A. (2004). The incidence of frontotemporal lobar degeneration in Rochester, Minnesota, 1990 through 1994. *Neurology, 62,* 606-508.

Launer, L. J., Andersen, K., Dewey, M. E., Letenneur, L., Ott, A., Amaducci, L. A., Copeland, J. R., Dartigues, F. F., Kragh-Sorensen, P., Martinez-Lage, J. M., Stijnen, T., & Hofman, A. (1999). Rates and risk factors for dementia and Alzheimer's disease: results from EURODEM pooled analyses. EURODEM Incidence Research Group and Work Groups. European Studies of Dementia. *Neurology, 52*(1), 78–84. doi:10.1212/wnl.52.1.78

Manly, J. J., & Mayeux, R. (2004). Ethnic differences in dementia and Alzheimer's disease. In N. B. Anderson, National Research Council (U.S.), R. A. Bulatao, & B. Cohen (Eds.), *Critical perspectives on racial and ethnic differences in health in late life* (pp. 95–141). National Academies Press.

Mehta, K. M., & Yeo, G. (2019). Incidence and prevalence of dementia in U.S. race and ethnic populations. In G. Yeo, L. Gerdner, & D. Gallagher-Thompson (Eds.), *Ethnicity and the dementias* (3rd ed., pp. 3–20). Routledge.

Paying for Senior Care. (2019, July 11, 2019). *Activities & instrumental activities of daily living—definitions, importance and assessment.* https://www.payingforseniorcare.com/activities-of-daily-living

Perkins, P., Annegers, J. F., Doody, R. S., Cooke, N., Aday, L., & Vernon, S. W. (1997). Incidence and prevalence of dementia in a multiethnic cohort of municipal retirees. *Neurology, 49*(1), 44–50. doi:10.1212/wnl.49.1.44

Pick, A., Girling, D. M., & Berrios, G. E. (1997). On the symptomatology of left-sided temporal lobe atrophy [Classic Text No. 29] (D. M. Girling & G. E. Berrios, Trans.). *History of Psychiatry, 8*(29, Pt 1), 149–159. doi:10.1177/0957154X9700802910

Plassman, B. L., Khachaturian, A. S., Townsend, J. J., Ball, M. J., Steffens, D. C., Leslie, C. E., Tschanz, J. T., Norton, M. C., Burke, J. R., Welsh-Bohmer, K. A., Hulette, C. M., Nixon, R. R., Tyrey, M., & Breitner, J. C. S. (2006). Comparison of clinical and neuropathologic diagnoses of Alzheimer's disease in 3 epidemiologic samples. *Alzheimer's & Dementia, 2*(1), 2–11. doi:10.1016/j.jalz.2005.11.001

Plassman, B. L., Langa, K. M., Fisher, G. G., Heeringa, S. G., Weir, D. R., Ofstedal, M. B., Burke, J. R., Hurd, M. D., Potter, G. G., Rodgers, W. L., Steffens, D. C., Willis, R. J., & Wallace, R. B. (2007). Prevalence of dementia in the United States: The aging, demographics, and memory study. *Neuroepidemiology, 29*(1–2), 125–132. doi:10.1159/000109998

Rocco, T. S. (2005). *From disability to critical race theory: Working towards critical disability theory* [Paper presentation]. Adult Education Research Conference, Athens GA. https://newprairiepress.org/aerc/2005/papers/17/

Schoenberg, B. S., Anderson, D. W., & Haerer, A. F. (1985). Severe dementia: Prevalence and clinical features in a biracial US population. *Archives of Neurologoy, 42*(8), 740–743. doi:10.1001/archneur.1985.04210090004002

Tang, M. X., Cross, P., Andrews, H., Jacobs, D. M., Small, S., Bell, K., Merchant, C., Lantigua, R., Cossta, R., Stern, Y., & Mayeux, R. (2001). Incidence of AD in African-Americans, Caribbean Hispanics, and Caucasians in northern Manhattan. *Neurology, 56*(1), 49–56. doi:10.1212/wnl.56.1.49

Valois, L., & Galvin, J. E. (2014). The role of the family in the care and management of patients with dementia. In B. Dickerson & A. Atri (Eds.), *Dementia: Comprehensive principles and practice* (pp. 609–621). Oxford University Press.

Chapter 4

Mixing Critical Qualitative Methods: Autoethnography and Phenomenology

Deconstructed Autoethnography

Autoethnography is a researcher's tool used to record, interpret, and analyze personal meanings from life experiences that provide explanations of personal, social, political, and cultural (Ellis, 2004) intersections. It's an evolving process and craft. Situated Positional Intersectionality (Figure 4.1) theorizes autoethnography as supported by my life story (Linde, 1993) and reveals what is necessary for the reader to know about me (Linde, 2015) and what has positioned me for my role as my wife's caregiver. Constructions that form my life story are represented in Figure 4.1 and include the inner core of autobiography and the outer domain of autoethnography (Collins, 2008). When the autobiography and autoethnography parts are isolated, distinct meanings emerge. When the parts are integrated into a whole, however, deeper meanings and connections of the parts form a larger context of my life-story narrative. Each of these constructions is explored in this chapter.

Figure 4.1. *Situated Positional Intersectionality*

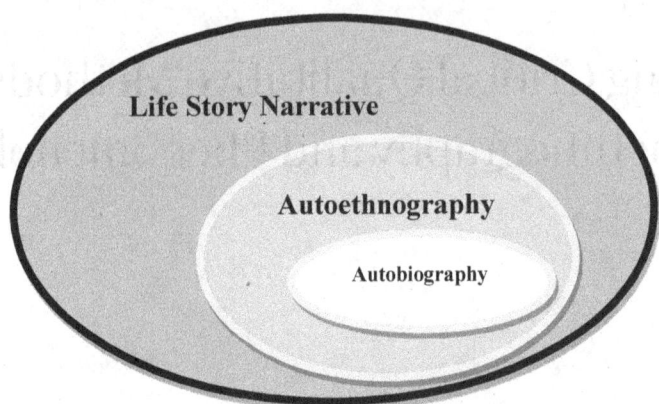

Source: Adapted from "Educational Differences: The Educational Backdrop of the Black Students of the 1954 Era and the Realities Of Contemporary African American Students," by D. R. Collins, 2008, *National FORUM of Multicultural Issues Journal, 5*(1), 1–22.

What Forms My Life Story?

Drawing from Urie Bronfenbrenner's (Broderick & Blewitt, 2020) ecological systems theory, my life story is affected by every experience in my life. From this large narrative, multiple narratives have emerged. The narratives presented in this book are parts of my grand narrative and are those of who I was, who I am, and who I will be. Although linear in nature, the only clear presentation is in the past. Interpretation of the present and future, then, is nebulous at best. The collective narrative presented throughout this book represents my life story. This narrative memory is thematic in nature (Linde, 2015). It is based on experiences that, at first, burst forth operantly, adding to existing ones to make sense of my life. Derived factors I identified in this collective recall include my developmental stages, social experiences, and actors in these. In contrast to unwritten reminders, written reminders tap into memories that provide context that include dates, times, settings, and actors. Some have been, but many have not been, recorded. The sounds of my voice, my body, and my relationships represent my complex life story. Unless I tell someone or write about them, they just happen to be. Their being is intertwined in my development spanning from my Black boyhood to my proud Black manhood. If I have not told anyone or written about them, they are floating personal memories at risk of being lost unless attached to a social and cultural context. These experiences include people throughout my life who have shown me love, attention, kindness, compassion, gentleness, patience, and a listening ear. It also encompasses people who have shown me hate, racism, and/or indifference; who did not see me; who have shown me evilness; and those who did not listen to me or denied me my voice. These experiences might have never been recorded. And even though I have had the hedge of protection from many harms, witnessing the hurt, harm, and inhumane acts suffered by family, friends, or strangers has been like enduring them firsthand. It, hurt or the perceived hurt of others, has engendered critical consciousness (Freire, 1970) in me that has been nurtured by my faith, my parents, and my wife early in our relationship. None of these experiences occurred in a vacuum but include actors in my life's story. They remain unrecorded fragile recollections until they are collected from memory and written.

Which comes first, memory or narrative?

Similar to the chicken-or-egg paradox, the dilemma of determining if memory or narrative came first or if one caused the other, depends on perspective. An argument could be made that narrative could not exist without the vessel of memory. On the other hand, when does memory start? A body of research on childhood amnesia suggests that memories can be recovered from as early as 1 year old (Robinson-Riegler & Robinson-Riegler, 2016). Embedded in these memories is context. Is the context the same as narrative? My wife often told me and others that at six months old, she remembers her parents having a party and standing up in her crib as people came into her bedroom to see her for the first time, to which I (even though I had never given any thought to memory at the time) and others, hearing this for the first time, gave her askance looks. Nonetheless, she offered as proof a picture of her all dressed up in one of those puffy baby dresses. She recounts that she remembers the flash when her mother took the picture. Despite initial suspicions, whenever my wife told this story, it was always consistently told, thereby eventually seeming credible. The bigger narrative in my wife's story was the depth of her memory or recall ability. Linde (2015) suggests that this "narrative is a representation, or a construction, based on a sequence of events in the past, that communicates something from the memory of the narrator" (p. 2) Linde further suggests that the memory resource can be, as in my wife's memory, supported by a photo representing a social context.

Analogous to the resource photo mentioned earlier are my personal journals, which provide context, and diary-type recollections of phenomenological memories. Selected journals' content represents memories for this book that focuses on my life story as a caregiver for my wife. Philosophically, from these memories that, in part, seem suspended in time but are collectively across time in a rectilinear fashion, I can construct a narrative of caregiving. Over time, my memories alone change due to maturity and attrition. In terms of maturity, for example, having children has given me clarity that I might not have understood previously to any great degree. In terms of attrition, Linde makes a point that "memory in narrative is necessarily social" (Linde, 2015, p. 1) This has become apparent to me as I recall life-story events.

On the way to biography or autobiography, my life story of existence is recorded in social artifacts (photographs, birth certificate, baptismal record, marriage license, shot record, school records, etc.) that represent my personhood. Additionally, personal journals help to solidify narratives from memories.

What forms my autobiography?

Surrounded by autoethnography, autobiography (Gibbs, 2018; Smith, 1998) reveals my voice as caregiver (Smith, 2013). Dissecting (Gibbs, 2018) the word *autobiography*, *auto* refers to me or the self, *bio–* refers to about me or my experiences, and *–graph*, my writings about me and my experiences that form my story or narrative. Moreover, these (*auto-bio-graphy*) also provide a lens through which to interpret experiences in life. It is in biography (not represented in Figure 4.1) or autobiography that my life story is written or documented. My autobiography exemplifies distinctiveness. For the most part, neither of these requires citations because they are written about or by a person and, unless the person is living by someone else's playbook, are original. Its particularity may describe my childhood, family, culture, and experiences within these. Words capture the phenomena of my life and emerge as my grand narrative, representing my life but not all of it. All of it could never be captured in words. This narrative is but an attempt to describe life occurrences. Words emanate in an effort to capture the essence of my experiences. Although powerful, little or big words reduce my big experiences.

As I piece together my story, it sometimes seems to take on a life of its own jumping from topic to topic. The need to bridle my runaway thoughts becomes evident in my attempts to focus, but this slows and stifles the fluidity of my thoughts. The only way to rein in these thoughts is to make a note and come back to it. Returning to these thoughts, however, sometimes results in less inspiration about the idea. Maybe it's the excitement I experience in my attempt to capture my fluid thoughts that are unequal to my penning them. These thoughts are difficult to extract from my rapid fluid thought because of their metaphysical properties.

What forms my caregiver autoethnography? My collective written story is entrenched in my memory and journals and occurs in the presence of my wife. In this form, meaning and sense are explored. Gibbs (2018) draws from autoethnography scholars (Chang, 2016; Ellis et al., 2011; Whitinui, 2014) to elucidate the meanings of *auto-*, referring to me or self; *ethno-*, referring to my ethos and insider status (Banks, 2006; Jones et al., 2016); and *-graphy*, referring to my writings about me and my experiences that form my narrative. Autoethnography represents expressions in a broad culturally latent context during specific periods that include my biography and autobiography within my life story.

As the prefix *auto-* and the suffix *-graphy* were addressed earlier, the focus now turns to the root *ethno-*. Although not addressed here, the prefix and suffix of the new word have fresh, nuanced cultural meanings in the changed word. As *ethno-* has replaced *bio-* from *autobiography* to create *autoethnography*, a question to consider is, "Does *ethno-* exclude *bio-* in the new form?" As I deeply ponder meanings, I visualize *bio-* to represent my wardrobe of clothing. Figuratively speaking, I see *ethno-* to be dressed in street, play, work, Sunday clothes, or maybe even in after-five attire. Growing up, I remember my parents dressing up to go out, to church, to special events. I remember seeing my seamstress mother sitting at her sewing machine almost daily during my childhood. As my siblings and I grew older, I recall my mother sewing less, except to teach my sister how to sew; while I was in college, to make my aunt's wedding dress; and, later, to make flower girl dresses for my wedding. My dad played a role in making sure we shined our shoes Saturday night for church on Sunday. Even though he did not accompany us to church on many Sundays, it was a reverent day for my dad in that we could not do things like mow the yard or work on our bicycles or do work in the garage. Returning to the question of whether *ethno-*, clothes for different occasions, includes *bio-*, the wardrobe of clothes, I suggest that it does.

Culture, the *ethno–* in *autoethnography*, is a complex interpretive grounding that intersects not only with the self and the written but also broadly with the cultural components of "shared values, practices, and social norms and worldviews associated with a particular cultural group" (Hays & McLeod, 2018, p. 5). In novel fashion, my worldview lens has shifted to accommodate my new real ontological perspectives in the landscape of triple grief (Maddrell, 2015), husband caregiving, fatherhood, and, despite my resistance, adulthood. Peeling back other layers of my cultural group components, racial discrimination, elements of faith, race, ethnicity, gender, Black middle-class status, caregiving, and baby-boomer status are revealed. And, under each of these components, multiple sub-elements reveal deeper insights and quandaries.

Race (Cameron & Wycoff, 1998) and ethnicity (Phinney, 1996) are complex and highly debated concepts and are often confused with the other. I identify as a light-skinned racially Black male. My wife identifies as a brown-skinned racially Black female. Our racial features refer to our characteristics, including skin color and the shape of our noses and eyes (Cameron & Wycoff, 1998; Zuckerman, 1990) that signify our African descent. Race is socially constructed and manipulated for individual, political, and psychological selections and motivations (Hays & McLeod, 2018). While our race refers to our physical characteristics, constructions, and descent, our ethnicity refers to cultural characteristics.

Ethnically, my wife and I identify as African Americans because of shared cultural group customs and social norms (Hays & Shillingford-Butler, 2018). Included in these are our belief systems, work ethic, Christian faith, genders, sexual orientations, African American middle-class status, baby-boomer generational ties, and language.

Caregiver Husband Status. The diagnosis of early-onset dementia for my wife expanded our cultural experiences exponentially. Specifically, by the nature of my wife's experience as having dementia, caregiver was added to my cultural experiences as well. My role has progressively changed to provide care 24 hours, 7 days a week. The change from taking care of only myself and sharing the care of our children to providing direct care to my wife for all her activities of daily living has caused a shift in every aspect of my life. Early on after the diagnosis, minimal caregiving evolved to moderate to total caregiving. Most of the time, I attend to all my wife's needs. Our daughter makes herself available to care for her mother any time and to provide respite to me several days weekly. This respite allows me to go into my office and accomplish other work-related activities. We also bring an attendant in two to three times a week to usually allow me to do our weekly shopping. Although we have an extensive network of family and friends who have offered to provide whatever care we need, we have not accepted their generous offers.

Physically, providing total care is exhausting. My wife has gone from walking to needing to be transported by wheelchair to different locations in and out of our house. Lifting has become a major part of caregiving.

Emotionally, a huge burden to me is double grieving, watching my wife daily lose cognitive ability along with the loss of her physical abilities and the unshakable reality that this incurable disease will eventually take her life. Unshakable, too, is the bereavement I feel for the loss of our son, which compounds into triple grieving, which I talk about later.

As the disease has progressed, my wife has become nonverbal. This means she cannot tell us what hurts, when she needs to go to the bathroom, or when she is hungry. As a caregiver, and with great difficulty, I must anticipate my wife's needs and strive to meet them.

With early consultation with our doctors, we decided we would maintain my wife at home. Fortunately, and because we have insurance, we are able to bring into our home doctors, nurses, and occupational and physical therapists. Additionally, doctor office visits occur on a regular basis and necessitate our going to their respective offices.

Data Collection/Life Journaling

Dialectically, autoethnography and phenomenology are based on lived experiences. Data emergence is constant (Van Manen, 2016), occurring every day, minute by minute. While Martin and Nakayama (1999) theorized relational dialectical theory to explore intercultural relationships of diverse people (Boylorn & Orbe, 2014), I draw on the theory to understand the complexities of a mixed-methods approach to my life as caregiver to my wife.

The Experiential Nature of Writing Autoethnography: Serendipity

A method of analysis I use in autoethnography is experiential writing. While I appreciate and was taught well the process of coding, sorting, and categorizing to the emergent theme, it is not the analysis process I utilize here. That process, however, is probably foundational to my understanding of qualitative analysis. The analysis I allowed to flow was emergent (Richardson & St. Pierre, 2005). It is an analysis method Elizabeth Adams St. Pierre (2005b) describes as, "*Thought happened in the writing. . . . I watched word after word appear. . . . I had not thought before I wrote them*" (p. 970, emphasis in original). The intentional, unintentional, intentional nature of this genre of writing yields serendipitous awareness. Like Robert Frost's (1915) poem, "The Road Not Taken," writing autoethnography is not straightforward but divergent. Learnings and realizations from experiences make life stories complex and unique. Through this experiential analysis, messy, scattered thoughts are organized as I take unforeseen paths that do not end but go on with embedded meanings. Journaling, my snippets of life, connect life to interpretation, significance, and purpose. During high school, I began to experience writing taking me on journeys. This became more apparent in college, and with attention from my English and writing teachers, I developed skills in writing. One encouraging experience I recall was from an unlikely source. The source was the dean of English. A strategy he used was to have his students read their papers in scheduled writing sessions. I had avoided taking classes from him because he was the dean. In my mind, I felt threatened that my vulnerabilities in writing would be exposed. When I finally met with him, almost immediately I felt at ease talking with him and reflected on my avoidance of him until I was forced to take his class in my senior year. He shared his early teaching experiences and told me I should go to graduate school and earn a doctorate. Although this was the farthest idea for me at the time, I attribute my ultimate pursuit of my doctorate to this encounter. As I read my paper about my experience as a young child watching my mother eat yogurt, finish dressing, and drive with her knee across town to teach, my professor told me he felt like he was in the car too. I kept waiting for the fictional "Ms. Fiddish" who made a big deal out of the most minuscule writing error. She never showed. More than that, he guided me in a discussion about my mother's tenacity. It was here I learned about the power of experience. And, although I don't remember anything particularly experiential about this writing, exploring writing for knowings took root. As I have written about this experience over time, meanings, such as clarified career paths and understandings, have emerged anew.

In my last undergraduate English class focusing on pedagogy, my college professor discussed with us how to use David Kolb's (1975) experiential learning theory to explore our students' experiences to interest them in writing. At the time, the theory was just another one to learn about and fortunately, to practice in context, although of minor significance until I began to attempt to teach students to write. In my first job as a high school English teacher and yet not recalling the theory, I found students excited with experiential prompts. Similarly, at the college level, I found it motivational to start with experiential writing and to make connections to other writing genres. As a result, students' writing skills improved. At the graduate level, I continue to observe the benefit of students' experiential writing on research topics of their interests.

Phenomenology Within Autoethnography

Bearings in Phenomenology

Phenomenology, in terms of this book, is the study and attention to my lived experiences of caregiving to my wife who experiences dementia. Phenomenology emanated early in the 20th century from Edmund Husserl (Zahavi, 2003), a German philosopher. Beyond Husserl, other selected historical and contemporary philosophers of phenomenology, who engaged in complex peer associations and rhetoric that I draw meaning from include (but are not limited to) Frantz Fanon (1925–1961) and Maurice Merleau-Ponty (1908–1961; Mahendran, 2007), Jean-Paul Sartre (1905–1980; Martinot, 2020), W. E. B. Du Bois (1868–1963) (DuBois, 1903, 1933; McAuley, 2020; Morris, 2017), and Jacques Derrida (1930-2004) (Armstrong, 1979). Other philosophers I draw meaning from include, Karl Marx (1818-1883), Booker T. Washington (1856-1915), Paul Laurence Dunbar (1872-1906), Carter G. Woodson (1875-1950), Mary McLeod Bethune (1875-1955), Marcus Garvey (1887-1940), Martin Luther King, Jr. (1919-1968), Malcolm X (1925-1965), Audre Lorde (1934-1992), Angela Davis (1944-), James Baldwin (1947-1987), Gloria Watkins, AKA bell hooks (1952-), Cornel West (1953-), and many others.

As a method, phenomenology is grounded in living the caregiver experience as I explore my wife's objective medical condition from a subjective perspective. Also, objective are the caregiver tasks, as described in Chapter 5, that must be done daily to provide my wife with a quality of living and to sustain her life. In essence the act of performing caregiving arises from my wife's needs as a result of dementia, a medical phenomenon.

Below I explore aspects of caregiving that are expressed as overlapping philosophical assumptions (Creswell & Poth, 2018) that connect reality (ontology), knowledge (epistemology), values (axiology) and interpretive analysis (methodology). Interpretive analyses are provided as autoethnography and phenomenography methodologies are explored throughout this book. These assumptions provide bearings to the overall phenomenon as laid out in my autoethnography.

Ontological Bearings. Ontologically (Anderson, 2014), as my wife's condition is a reality, so is my caregiving. This caregiver reality is absorbed in concern questions about suffering. Specifically, I question, *is she suffering?* if so, *to what extent?* and *what can I do to take the suffering away or reduce it? I know that she experiences pain as a result of excessive sitting, since her muscles are atrophying because of advanced dementia. What emotional and mental suffering is she experiencing?* So as I perceive her suffering, I suffer. In essence the act of performing caregiving arises from my wife's needs as a result of dementia. I am aware of options available to us that could place her away from our home, but my inner sense feels a viability of at-home care. After my wife and I talked after her diagnosis, she encouraged me to place her in a care facility so that I would not be tied to her when dementia was in its advanced stages. Our long talks after her diagnosis reminded me of our long talks before we had children. We had long talks when we were raising our children, but those talks involved either them or someone other than the two of us. These talks were more spiritual talks that we could have after working through our marriage, differences, and the list goes on. During these talks my wife told me she did not want to be a burden on me. Part of me felt she said this because she felt she had to. But, as time went on, she showed me pictures of memory care, nursing and other places on the internet, as though we were shopping for a house. At that, I knew she was serious. Since I could not get her to stop showing them to me, I would look at them and we even talked about them to appease her. In her wittiness, she asked me which one I wanted her to put me in. We had a big laugh. Each time I reminded her I could not place her in a nursing home unless I could not medically take care of her. On reflection, my inner self wanted to keep my wife near me. I had not thought it at the time, but I wanted new memories of her smiling, laughing. I wanted to look into her eyes every night and morning. I wanted to comfort her when she became anxious because of dementia and to take care of her needs, even though it is a struggle to always know what they are.

One issue we rarely talked about though was death, hers or mine. But because of a series of family deaths, it became a topic almost naturally. We buried our son near his maternal grandparents. At the grave site, I noticed there was only one plot left near him and my wife's parents. So I brought this to my wife's attention and asked her if she wanted me to purchase it for her so she could be buried near our son and her parents. She asked where I would be if she were buried there, and I told her I could be buried near my parents across town. I told her we could both be buried there. Too quickly, she decided to be buried near our son. So, we bought the plot nearest to him. I found the transaction to be surreal, as I had never bought cemetery plots. Both of our parents had their own plots. My parents had several, with a family tombstone, which I knew about, but in an effort not to tilt the balance of the forces in the universe, I never asked my parents about them. One of my brothers once told me he was not born when they were purchased. Anyway, I was surprised we were presented with documents like a deed for each plot. As a husband caregiver, reality is relative and ever changing.

Epistemological Bearings. Epistemologically (Audi, 2003), this autoethnography refers to my evolving knowledge about the phenomenon of caregiving for dementia. This autoethnography guaranteed me a built-in place close to my caregiver phenomenon. In autoethnography, we lived in the epistemological field and could not leave the site. Until my wife's diagnosis of dementia, I learned about dementia through formal means and at the periphery of others caring for individuals. Although some of my knowledge about caregiving is based on what I observed, much of my knowledge was based on generalized knowledge from similar impairments and behaviors and, for the most part, in clinical settings. None of the knowledge was based on providing care for 24 hours a day. Discussions with family and friends about the dementia my wife was experiencing helped me understand that I wanted to have firsthand knowledge of my wife's experiences and not receive this information secondhand.

An initial first response to my wife's diagnosis was to treat her as though she was sick. For a while, I enabled her dependence on me and our children, taking from her, her cherished independence that was fading too quickly. Her independence was something attractive to me about her since high school. But forgiving myself for my shortsightedness helped me understand that the overprotection came from a place of concern. None of us knew what to do. What we felt was that we needed to do something. We began treating her as though she was in the advanced stage of dementia and no longer capable of doing things for herself. In her subtle manner, she told all of us that she was capable of doing things like dressing herself, making our bed, bathing, and many other things. In our bedroom soon after her diagnosis, I attempted to help her tie her tennis shoes on and was rebuked, with her saying she could do it herself. I explained that I was trying to help her. She retorted, "I'll let you know when I need your help." That was my first lesson and admonition to give her space to not only do for herself but also to process what was happening to her. In a later talk, she confided in me that she felt like she was abandoning our family and that there was nothing she could do. I had rushed to tie her shoes because I saw her as ill. Regardless of the number of times I had tied her shoes in the past, this new season meant brought on complexities with the realization that my wife was not who she used to be and who she and I thought she would be. We started grieving that loss. And we both felt lost in maneuvering this new path. My wife viewed her new season with great trepidation, and she wanted to but did not know how to own this new reality. I shared with her that my view was the same: We would still grow old together. I told her that the only difference was that I would be taking care of her instead of her prophecy that she would be the one taking care of me. She laughed and knew we would be alright, and I think my wife was consoled with this knowledge.

Along my caregiving journey and in my mind, I felt the need to separate dementia from who my wife was. But as time progressed, particularly during the advanced season, dementia and my wife intertwined into my beloved companion.

Axiological Bearings. Axiologically (Findlay, 1974; Hart & Embree, 2013), as in the landscape of autoethnography, the author's qualities and values are presented throughout this book. These include my race and ethnic identity, gender, generational reference, and family and marital status, among others. Also in different parts of the book are insights into value-laden interpretations of multiple life experiences.

After my wife's diagnosis, we had to make decisions that were different than what we planned. Changes in my wife's behavior seemed minimal after the diagnosis. For the most part, during the early stage, our activities remained the same. We went out to dinner, to the movies, to church, to the grocery store, shopping, and out with friends. One of the few signs of dementia's toll on her at the time was she became fatigued from intense attention to making sense of conversations and the environment. Slowly, she preferred to stay home and with our children and me. She still wanted to go out but would tire almost immediately and want to go home. She no longer recognized many families and friends, seeing them as strangers, and these "new" people caused her to be anxious. Our children made my role easy. I was able to go to work while they stayed at home with their mother. At that time, she sensed we were "hanging" around the house to watch her, and we were. Although at the early diagnosis stage, we felt comfortable leaving her alone for short periods, no longer than an hour. Her biggest problem at the time was boredom. She no longer had the freedom to go for a walk alone. The few times she did, she got lost but found her way back home. Getting lost created an anxiety that caused her to restrict venturing out alone. Our son walked with her most days afterward. Boredom is a complaint of many people who experience dementia. Out of concern that she would venture out again and get lost, we put bells on the ground-floor doors. Most of the time I monitored my wife, but when I went to work, one of our children stayed at home with her. This round-robin care worked for years until our son passed. Because his death was traumatic, additional complexities emerged, and her grief compounded by dementia caused her to emotionally and cognitively deteriorate at a faster rate, almost overnight. This burst of complexities manifested in her attempting to leave our house in search of our son and other deceased family members without telling anyone. At that point, we added another caregiver and upgraded our alarm system to monitor my wife in most of the rooms in our house.

Out of concern for my wife, many of her friends offered to come and be with her, and many did. They, along with some of my friends, asked me if I had considered placing my wife in a memory facility or nursing home. Some of them were surprised when I told them I planned to keep my wife at home as long as I could, barring medical situations I could not manage. Some friends, meaning well, advised me that I should be sure to take care of myself. My response was always the same: "I will." A few of our friends told me that my wife would not know if I put her in a home. Around this time, I learned about another husband I did not know whose friends said the same thing to him and his response was that even if she did not know, he did. So I used his words and told them the same: "I would know."

Explanation of Phenomenology in Autoethnography

Turning to an explanation of phenomenology, Vagle (2018) provides a metaphoric description of phenomenology elucidated from different altitudes analogies. He provides a valuable tool in explaining theories, in general, and phenomenology, specifically, to students, as well as providing deeper philosophical insight. Vagle explains phenomenological philosophical underpinnings or bearings as being at 30,000 feet. From philosophy, methodological interpretive schematic or representation are unfolded at 10,000 feet. At ground level, the ultimate implementation and execution of the theory occur.

Comparatively, when I have flown from my home in Houston, Texas (about 50–80 ft elevation), to Aspen (about 8,000 ft) or Aspen Mountain (11,000 ft), Colorado, I have experienced symptoms of altitude sickness (ABC News, 2006) lasting a few hours upon arrival, but for some people, adjusting to the altitude has been known to last for 1 to 2 days. Altitude sickness occurs because locations like Aspen have less oxygen in the air than a city like Houston, which is about 50 to 90 feet above sea level (Schaper, 2017). Mild altitude sickness symptoms are like those of the common flu. For my wife and me, the shortness of breath, dizziness, and body aches were the most annoying. Interestingly, when my children accompanied me to Aspen, they complained of no effects from the high altitude. Of course, age and wellness seem to play a role in who experiences altitude sickness. The majority of people, however, do not report symptoms when changing altitudes.

I find parallels to Vagle's (2018) constructed levels of altitude metaphor to human travel experiences by air carrier and his intended connections to elevations that unravel theory and make clearer theoretical connections. First, most people travel by an air carrier to 30,000 feet. Although, through acclimation and wellness, mountain climbers have scaled to altitudes of 29,029 feet of Mount Everest. This feat is analogous to contact with a philosophy. Initially, at first exposure (30,000 ft), the theory seems complex, maybe unclear. But as we study the theory, the philosophy becomes clearer. As we become more familiar with the theory, the more transparent it becomes.

Along the way, we may come across interpretations of the theory and develop a better understanding of the meanings intrinsic to the theory.

Continuing my analogy to Vagle's (2018) altitude construct, when viewing theory from 10,000 feet from an airplane, we see the terrain. At this level in a plane, we can see vista views of familiar and unfamiliar forests, wetlands, communities, and buildings. If we are familiar with the location we are looking at, we may recognize specific edifices, our particular neighborhood, lakes, and even our house. At this level, Vagle suggests we may recognize as familiar those parts of the theory we've applied or come in contact with through our scholarship. But at this view are parts of the theory we have not explored and may want to make broader connections to. Descending figuratively from 30,000 feet with a knowledge level of "philosophical, ontological, and epistemological concepts, ideas, and issues" (Vagle, 2018, p. 5) to 10,000 feet, where representative distinctions of theoretical, idealistic, metaphysical, and interpretive knowledge form emerging beliefs and opinions that create a methodology. Basically, we see connections between the theory and a methodology.

Most exciting to me is the landing or ground level. It is here that a theory about a phenomenon meets practice. More important, the ground level is where my experiences are lived and constantly interpreted. We are able to test and change the theory applied to phenomenological qualitative spaces. We can change the application of a theory to a phenomenon at any of Vagle's levels. At this level, however, we can experience the implementation of a theory firsthand. Physically, at ground level, our views are only limited to as far as we can see in a 360° rotation around the central axis of our body. When we make this rotation at ground level, however, we end up in the same location we started from with our visual perspective facing the place we started from. So, as we rotate, we have multiple perspective opportunities that by full rotation, we may enhance our 360° experience as far as we can see. But we are still limited by our ground level restriction. Moving our perspectives or visual reference to a higher level, our views, if unrestricted, enhance our point of reference, although still limited to ground level. Moving back down, we return to our ground-level perspective, although it might have been changed because of the experience of other viewpoints. So, even if we return to ground level, we may have broadened our perspective, thereby enhancing our understanding of a theory.

The ground level may be analogous to perspectives we can access through books. For example, from reading or hearing about a place, we may create a vision of this faraway place, but we are limited by what we read and possibly imagine. Our experience of reality of the place we read about is enhanced by visiting the actual place.

When Autoethnography Reveals Phenomenological Agony

I called on your name, LORD, FROM the depths of the pit.
You heard my plea: "Do not close your ears to my cry for relief."
You came near when I called you, and you said, "Do not fear."
You, Lord, took up my case; you redeemed my life.
                                            LAMENTATIONS 3:55–58 NIV

This chapter explores the components of autoethnography that may be not only evocative and empirical but also emotionally painful. In fact, as I presented a paper on agony revealed through autoethnography, at the 14th International Congress of Qualitative Inquiry in 2018, I became overwhelmed with emotion to the point of sobbing and barely getting through my paper. Before presenting my paper, I had read it several times without reaction when talking about my son's death in the context of taking care of my wife who is experiencing dementia. I felt I should be embarrassed but was not. I didn't have room for shame. My cup of emotion was spilling over. I had attended but had not presented at the conference since my son's death.

Through a critical qualitative inquiry lens, a narrative that illustrates self-reflection on personal experiences is constructed and results in a deeper awareness by engaging with the inquisitive subject. Explored are the individual, personal, and subjective interpretations of firsthand experiences. Drawing from grounded theory (Glaser & Strauss, 1967), through systematic collection, phenomena may be validated by analysis and interpretation.

Important key terms in this chapter are the following: *Autoethnography* refers to the introspective. *Critical qualitative inquiry* refers to complex lived experiences with meanings on multiple levels of analysis. *Narrative* refers to a lived experience with known and or unknown meanings. *Critical agony* refers to profound trauma and observed and experienced debilitating affliction.

Lived Grief Experiences

Grief has new meanings to me. On the one hand it is the loss of the mind of the woman of my life and dreams to the debilitating affliction of dementia. In the midst of my wife's cognitive struggles, and on the other hand is the complication of our son, Cody, taking his life. It continues with what seems to be an overnight display of psychosis that manifested in delusions by my wife of our son visiting our new next-door neighbors, even though we buried him the previous week. The psychosis is compounded with auditory and visual hallucinations of my wife's deceased mother and father also visiting our neighbors along with our son. She is determined to go and see them and goes out the front door in her pajamas, housecoat, and house shoes. I convince her to come back to the house by telling her we'll go and visit them after we get dressed. I am terrified of our neighbors' reaction to her if she ever made it to their front door. She continues to plan these visits over the course of the next few weeks. This new terror causes my daughter and me to contact my wife's doctor. She immediately prescribed my wife an antipsychotic that controlled the wandering behavior. She commented to me that she was surprised my wife had not experienced psychosis earlier. Prior to this episode and at every visit after her diagnosis, the doctor asked me if my wife had seen people who were not present and each time, I informed her I had not observed delusions until now.

When Grief Calls

My previous experience with dementia had been in clinical settings where I worked professionally with multiple dementia patients for brief periods. And even though it was not a focus of my study, I wrote a major paper on the topic of dementia in my master's counseling program. But this did not prepare me for the 24/7 care of managing my wife's activities of daily living. And now, beyond intersectionality, my grief was intertwined with death, daily cognitive decline, and my wife's impending physical death. The three seemed inseparable and the sum of gloom.

A critical examination of lived phenomena related to grief due to the death of my son and the ostensible exacerbation of dementia of my wife culminated in emotional expression that just was. Typically, I publicly avoided triggers of sobbing, but at the Qualitative Congress, in the moment, reading of the words caught me off guard. This was my new reality, and it permeated all aspects of my life. It was the type of phenomena that Ellis (2016) says she often writes about and "knock[s] her off her feet" (p. 34). My agony with triple grief was a new phenomenon for me. I had lost many loved ones and attended many funerals. While my faith provided me the greatest comfort, its mystery unnerved me.

Still, until my cumulative losses, prolonged bereavement seemed distant to me, something others experienced that touched them directly but was always at bay with me. It had been a spectator event. I constantly prayed that my son was not sentenced to eternal damnation for taking his life. As I searched my life's faith, I could not find any time or anyone who told me that suicide resulted in one's soul being lost. But in all my informal and formal religious and faith training, I could not find a definitive answer to my question of whether my boy would go to heaven or hell for taking his life. I could not remember a conversation with either my mother or father or anyone who stated that suicide resulted in eternal damnation. I understood that biblical death meant a figurative death to Jesus. This must be a socialized belief I internalized that tormented my soul. My soul could not find comfort.

I relied on my mother when my father passed and my wife when my mother passed, but she was now no longer emotionally available to comfort me in grieving the daily loss of her due to dementia and the loss of our son. I found I had no construct for dealing with this kind of grief. I will say that, at the time of our son's suicide, I felt God by my side, and this gave me peace as I wandered through the aftermath. Not recognizing it at the time, my faith was being tested and I was having what Cynthia Dillard (2008) termed "The Blessing of Clarity" (p. 82) in my spiritual faith through this grief, even though my soul was not at peace. As Ellis (2004) offers, new meanings of loss emerged. Beyond this, I also experienced effects I was surprised to acknowledge. Before my cumulative experience, I would have intellectualized the new feeling as numbness. But I recognized it as something more. I am still not sure of what it is, but it has emerged as a result of tremendous and ongoing loss—not the total loss Job of the Bible experienced because I still had health and many of the people and possessions stripped from Job. But then again, it felt like a total loss to me. But what was "it?" While I still don't know, I recognize new complexities and dispositions such as feeling at ease with a new normal of being in the state of grief. Paxton (2018) describes in his book, titled *At Home With Grief: Continued Bonds With the Deceased*, his experience with this phenomenon. Paxton tells an enlightening story of the bonds before and after his mother's death. Being at ease with grief was a new phenomenon, as my training as a counselor taught me to help people move on from grief. Not moving "on" and feeling a seemingly permanent dark malaise seemed unnatural, but comforting, to me.

This comfort may be akin to what Maddrell (2015) characterizes as a "normal response" (p. 168) to significant death. I agree with Maddrell in her assertion that the loss of my son felt like a snatching from my core. Because of the mental connections and triggered remembrances, the loss is held in, in what Maddrell, taken from Rohr (2002), describes as a "sacred place" (2015, p. 168) in me. This place holds memories that may only be tapped when the loss is so intimate and primitive that there is no space in our culture for separating or distancing ourselves from reality. Information revealed through journaling and reflection form and represent this in life narratives. While the autoethnographic technique allowed cultural exploration, the phenomenological tool of separating and bracketing loss, in a counseling sense (Kocet & Herlihy, 2014), seemed unavailable to me. Multiple personal perspectives were explored through the use of life-story narrative, autoethnography, and autobiography. In the life-story autobiographies, the subject and author's writings reflect relationships in the family unit. The exploration takes an autoethnography perspective in which the author provided personal self-reflection to meanings in the family milieu. As shown in Figure 4.2, an emerging visual relational perspective of the "self-in-relation-to-others" (Hernandez & Ngunjiri, 2013) allows visual analysis that seeks to explore lived experiences perceived by the husband caregiver to his wife and their daughter that is complicated by their son taking his life. Reflections on relational phenomena provide the autoethnographic introspection. Introspection seeks to study the meaning of a phenomenon revealed within the context of this agonizing setting. Reflective journaling and observations seek to understand if and how shared experiences transcend multiple contexts. The inquiry further seeks to objectively distinguish what is expressed and expected and what is not expressed. Subjectively, the inquiry seeks introspective connections between reflections and stories.

Figure 4.2. *Emerging Visual Relational Perspective*

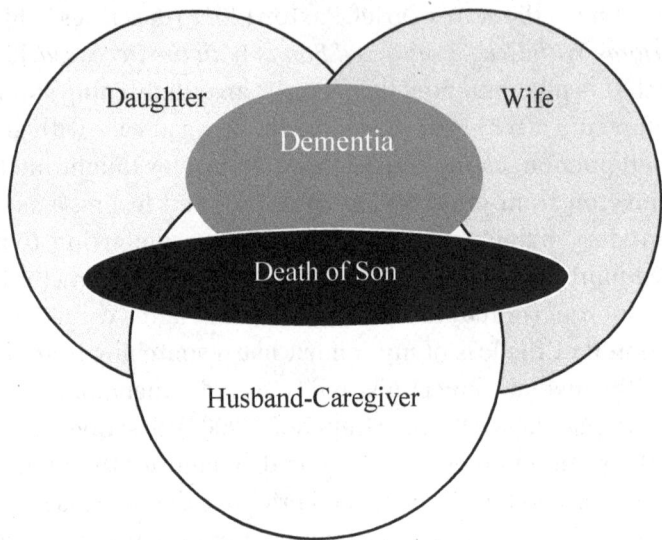

Ineffable Eidetic Knowings

Autoethnography is the ultimate insider expression. Everyone else is an outsider. Personal experience is constantly generating thoughts, meanings, actions, and reactions. Paradoxical is the experience of thought and meaning. Even if we accept that thought may come before experience, separating the two is complex and circular. Furthermore, as raised in Chapter 6, how does language or words emerge from thought and experience? I perceive thought to be superior, even mystical, to language and, as such, reduced in written form. I am not suggesting that the written word is not powerful, but I am suggesting individual's thinking cannot be matched and to do so is to lessen the original conscience perception. And it must be acknowledged that writing about stressful events has positive mental and physical outcomes (Pennebaker & Francis, 2010). This level of thought seeks to connect the event to language, thereby lessening the wandering "ante-predictive life of consciousness" (Merleau-Ponty, 1962, p. iv). Autoethnography is more than a written recording; it is the result of a series of conscious thoughts that have resulted in understanding the meanings of experiences. In my case, the experience meanings are embodied in caregiving to my wife. By definition, autoethnography must be written; otherwise, it is incomprehensible, illiterate.

As I read Maddrell's (2015) article "Mapping Grief: A Conceptual Framework for Understanding the Spatial Dimensions of Bereavement, Mourning and Remembrance," I was reminded of the meaning of the word *ineffable* (p. 169) and its contextual meaning, "unspeakable." Focusing on "unspeakable," my recollection of this scarcely seen or used word by me was its use in trauma literature. Before looking it up again, I thought its primary definition, "disgusting or awful," did not reflect its deeper meanings. I thought the former represented a "disgusting" act or "awful" experience, like the murder of George Floyd by Minneapolis police on May 25, 2020.[1] From this travesty, the Black Lives Matter movement was set ablaze from smoldering embers of decades-long abuse and killings by police officers across the United States of primarily Black and Brown men. This act was not only ineffable because we saw the active killing of someone in prime time, but it was eidetic (Van Manen, 2016, pp. 228–230). Witnessing Mr. Floyd's murder and then trying to speak it is what Van Manen, using "Husserlian reduction proper," describes an eidetic reduction (2016, p. 229). Eidetically, I would never need to see it again and would remember it forever because I could, before engaging in reflection, describe factually, although not completely, the phenomenon witnessed. My visceral reflection has shaped my lived experience but may not be able to form my complete thinking about the experience (Merleau-Ponty, 1962) in Van Manen (2016). In effect, I may seek to bracket (in the Husserlian sense) the eidetic process because the "saturated phenomenon" is unspeakable, deficient in word articulation, but apparent in my phenomenological social consciousness. Returning to my exploration of the word *ineffable*, its meaning to me is in relation to my experience with grief on multiple levels. The connotation of the word is surreal in its mystery. But elevating feeling to fluid thought to an articulated level, even though eventually necessary, reduces the experience.

---

1 George Floyd was killed when Derek Chauvin kept his knee on his neck for 9 minutes 29 seconds, after being handcuffed and held down by three other officers, at the direction of Chauvin. Mr. Floyd repeated, "I can't breathe," to no avail. Recognizing his impending death, Mr. Floyd called for his deceased mother. Mr. Floyd was taken unresponsive to the hospital where he was pronounced dead. His murder was recorded by a passerby and broadcast to the world.

Reader Thought Questions and Further Reading

1. How did the author deconstruct autoethnography?
2. What is the role of writing in autoethnography?
3. How does memory inform the narrative?
4. How does the author form his caregiver autoethnography?
5. How are the concepts of "experiential writing" and "serendipity" connected?
6. Differentiate ontological, epistemological, axiological, and methodological bearings and their significance in the chapter.
7. What is the significance of the altitude analogy to theory?
8. How is agony revealed as a phenomenon in autoethnography?
9. What is the significance of grief in a lived narrative presented in the chapter?
10. Why is the visual relational perspective emerging?

References

ABC News. (2006, January 6). *The air up there*. https://abcnews.go.com/Business/FlyingHigh/story?id=1041338&page=1

Anderson, V. (2014). Black ontology and theology. In K. G. Cannon & A. B. Pinn (Eds.), *The Oxford handbook of African American theology* (pp. 390–401). Oxford University Press.

Armstrong, E. G. (1979). Black sociology and phenomenological sociology. *The Sociological Quarterly, 20*(3), 387–397.

Audi, R. (2003). *Epistemology*. Routledge.

Banks, J. A. (2006). *Cultural diversity and education: Foundations, curriculum and teaching*. Pearson.

Boylorn, R. M., & Orbe, M. P. (2014). *Critical autoethnography: Intersecting cultural identities in everyday life*. Left Coast Press.

Broderick, P. C., & Blewitt, P. (2020). *The life span: Human development for helping professionals*. Pearson.

Cameron, S. C., & Wycoff, S. M. (1998). The destructive nature of the term race: Growing beyond a false pardigm. *Journal of Counseling & Development, 76*, 277–285.

Chang, H. (2016). Autoethnography in research: Growing pains? *Qualitative Health Research, 26*(4), 443–451.

Collins, D. R. (2008). Educational differences: The educational backdrop of the Black students of the 1954 era and the realities of contemporary African American students. *National FORUM of Muliticultural Issues Journal, 5*(1), 1–22.

Creswell, J., & Poth, C. N. (2018). *Qualitative inquiry research design* (4th ed.). Sage.

Dillard, C. B. (2008). A whole sense of self, a whole sense of the world: The blessings of spirituality in qualitative research and teaching. *International Review of Qualitative Research, 1*(1), 81–101.

Du Bois, W. E. B. (1903). *The souls of Black folk*. A. C. McClurg.

Du Bois, W. E. B. (1933). Marxism and the Negro problem. *The Crisis, 40*(5), 103–104, 118. http://www.webdubois.org/dbMNP.html

Ellis, C. (2004). *The ethnographic I: A methodological novel about autoethnography.* AltaMira Press.

Ellis, C., Adams, T. E., & Bochner, A. (2011). Autoethnography: An overview. *Forum: Qualitative Social Research, 12*(1), Article 10. https://www.qualitative-research.net/index.php/fqs/article/view/1589/3095

Jones, S. H., Adams, T., & Ellis, C. (2016). Coming to know autoethnography as more than a method. In S. H. Jones, T. E. Adams, & C. Ellis (Eds.). New York: Routledge.

Findlay, J. N. (1974). Axiological ethics. In W. D. Hudson (Ed.), *New studies in ethics.* Palgrave. https://doi.org/10.1007/978-1-349-02399-8_2

Freire, P. (1970). *Pedagogy of the oppressed*. Continuum.

Frost, R. (1915). The road not taken [Poem]. https://poets.org/poem/road-not-taken

Gibbs, A. (2018). Ethical issues when undertaking autoethnographic research with families. In R. Iphofen & M. Tolich (Eds.), *The SAGE handbook of qualitative reserch ethics* (pp. 148–160). Sage.

Glaser, B., & Strauss, A. L. (1967). *The discovery of grounded theory: Strategies for qualitative research*. Aldine.

Hart, J. G., & Embree, L. (Eds.). (2013). *Phenomenology of value and valuing* (Vol. 28). Springer.

Hays, D. G., & McLeod, A. L. (2018). The culturally competent counselor. In D. G. Hayes & B. T. Erford (Eds.), *Developing multicultural counseling competence: A systems approach* (3rd ed., pp. 2–36). Pearson.

Hays, D. G., & Shillingford-Butler, A. (2018). Racism and White privilege. In D. G. Hays & B. T. Erford (Eds.), *Developing multicultural counseling competence: A systems approach* (pp. 92–126). Pearson.

Hernandez, K.-A. C., & Ngunjiri, F. (2013). Relationships and comunnities in autoethnography. In S. H. Jones, T. E. Adams, & C. Ellis (Eds.), *Handbook of autoethnography* (pp. 262–280). Routledge.

Jones, S. H., Adams, T., & Ellis, C. (2016). Coming to know autoethnography as more than a method. In S. H. Jones, T. Adams, & C. Ellis (Eds.), *Handbook of autoethnography* (pp. 7–47). Routledge.

Kocet, M. M., & Herlihy, B. J. (2014). Addressing value-based conflicts within the counseling relationship: A decision-making model. *Journal of Counseling & Development, 92*(2), 180–186.

Kolb, D. A. (1975). Toward an applied theory of experiential learning. In C. Cooper (Ed.), *Theories of group processes* (pp. 33–57). John Wiley.

Linde, C. (1993). *Life stories: The creation of coherence.* Oxford University Press.

Linde, C. (2015). Memory in narrative. In K. Tracy, C. Ilie, & T. Sandel (Eds.), *The international encyclopedia of language and social interaction.* John Wiley & Sons. https://onlinelibrary.wiley.com/doi/pdf/10.1002/9781118611463.wbielsi121

Maddrell, A. (2015). Mapping grief: A conceptual framework for understanding the spatial dimensions of bereavement, mourning and remembrance. *Social and Cultural Geography, 17*(2), 166–188.

Mahendran, D. (2007). The facticity of Blackness: A non-conceptual approach to the study of race and racism in Fanon's and Merleau-Ponty's phenomenology. *Human Architecture: Jounal of the Sociology of Self-Knowledge, 5*(3). : http://scholarworks.umb.edu/humanarchitecture/vol5/iss3/18

Martin, J. N., & Nakayama, T. K. (1999). Thinking dialectically about culture and communication. *Communication Theory, 9*(1), 1–25. https://doi.org/10.1111/j.1468-2885.1999.tb00160.x

Martinot, S. (2020). *Sartre and the structure of White racialized identity.* https://www.ocf.berkeley.edu/~marto/sartre&wri.htm

McAuley, C. (2020, February 21). Max Weber and the souls of Black folk. *Church Life Journal.* https://churchlifejournal.nd.edu/articles/max-weber-and-the-souls-of-black-folk/

Merleau-Ponty, M. (1962). *Phenomenology of perception* (C. Smith, Trans.). Routledge and Kegan Paul.

Morris, A. (2017). W. E. B. Du Bois at the center: From science, civil rights movement, to Black Lives Matter. *The Bristish Journal of Sociology 68*(1), 3–16.

Paxton, B. (2018). *At home with grief.* Routledge.

Pennebaker, J. W., & Francis, M. E. (2010). Cognitive, emotional, and language processes in disclosure. *Cognition & Emotion, 10*(6), 601–626.

Phinney, J. S. (1996). When we talk about American ethnic groups: What do we mean? *American Psychologist, 51*(9), 918–927.

Richardson, L., & St. Pierre, E. A. S. (2005). Writing: A method of inquiry. In N. Denzin & Y. S. Lincoln (Eds.), *The SAGE handbook of qualitative research* (3rd ed.). Sage.

Robinson-Riegler, B., & Robinson-Riegler, G. L. (2016). *Cognitive psychology: Applying the science of the mind* (4th ed.). Pearson.

Rohr, R. (2002). Grieving as sacred space. *Sojourners Magazine*(31), 20-24. doi:https://sojo.net/magazine/january-february-2002/grieving-sacred-space

Schaper, D. (2017, August 31). *3 reasons Houston was a 'sitting duck' for Harvey flooding*. NPR. https://www.npr.org/2017/08/31/547575113/three-reasons-houston-was-a-sitting-duck-for-harvey-flooding

Smith, L. M. (1998). Biographical method. In N. K. Denzin & Y. S. Lincoln (Eds.), *Strategies of qualitative inquiry* (pp. 184–224). Sage.

Smith, L. M. (2013). Biographical method. In J. Goodwin (Ed.), *SAGE biographical research* (pp. 1–36). Sage.

Vagle, M. D. (2018). Crafting phenomenological research. Routledge.

Van Manen, M. (2016). *Phenomenology of practice: Meaning-giving methods in phenomenological research and writing*. Routledge.

Whitinui, P. (2014). Indigenous autoethnography: Exploring, engaging, experiencing "self" as a native method inquiry. *Journal of Contemporary Ethnography, 43*(4), 456–487.

Zahavi, D. (2003). *Husserl's phenomenology*. Stanford University Press.

Zuckerman, M. (1990). Some dubious premises in research and theory on racial differences: Scientific, social, and ethical issues. *American Psychologist, 45*(12), 1297–1303.

Chapter 5

• • • • • • • • •

Safely and Softly Up and Down the Staircase and Axiology

You are observing special days and months and seasons and years!
GALATIANS 4:10 NIV

This chapter explores the phenomenological within an autoethnographic narrative of climbing and descending stairs as synonymous to caregiving during the progression of my wife's dementia in a post-disability era. A nondirectional philosophical frame is supported by an axiological consciousness structure that intersects with historical African values, which include ontological and epistemological suppositions that further intersects with critical, critical race, and critical disability theories. From this analysis, I seek to gain insight by painting a narrative picture of drawing from participatory (Heron & Reason, 1997) theory as caregiver.

The Stairs—Avoiding Falls

A major priority I have is to help my wife avoid falls. As her gait has become more unstable, I now assist her in all of her standing and walking. I have witnessed the downward spiral of an elderly love one fall and hit his head on a stone counter. The National Council on Aging's (2020) Falls Prevention Program suggests strategies to help avoid falls. Escorting my wife around the house as she experiences the severe stage of dementia is a labor of love because of the time and energy it takes to ensure her safety. Treacherous places in our house include the bathrooms, the kitchen, and the stairs because of the hardwood and stone floors and countertops in these spaces. As a result of her increasingly impaired gait, we have removed all rugs and place them back when they are needed. Also, the dementia my wife experiences causes her to pinch and grab my or any caregiver's clothing, wrists, arms, or surfaces and objects she can access. This behavior makes it difficult to balance or steady her when standing, sitting, or moving her in her wheelchair or walker. When she tightly grabs my wrist, before moving, I must loosen her tight grasp by turning my wrist to where her thumb and fingers meet and execute a release. This tight grasp causes excruciating pain of my wrist, because of osteoarthritis in my wrists, necessitating a quick release. When possible, however, wearing a wristband helps in the avoidance of this pain. This release is similar to a defensive release taught in martial arts. This release usually occurs while I am using the other hand to balance her if she is standing. If she is sitting, I am able to use my other hand to aid my release. When she pinches clothing, hers or mine, care has to be taken to pull the clothing away without harming her, as her fingers are often tangled in the shirt, throw blanket, or bedding, for example. When she tightly grips a grab bar in the bathroom, care is taken to pry her fingers away without any harm to her. It seems that her tight grasp of anyone or anything is an attempt to steady herself, but this does not prevent her from losing her balance, as she has less control of her balance.

A fall anywhere is not good and, as with my loved one, can be tragic. The fact that our master bedroom is on the second level necessitates that I assist my wife in going up and down the stairs. Most days, my wife is sedentary. So standing, sitting, and walking to the bathroom or traversing the stairs is the most exercise she gets. On bad days, we stay upstairs. Bad days occur more often as the dementia progresses, but these are days when my wife is more confused. She moves slower, taking tiny steps, stopping often, and requiring more support. On some of these days, she might sit on her walker seat as I roll it from a recliner in the bedroom to the bathroom. Usually from the bathroom, I encourage her to walk back to the bedroom recliner, saying, "Walk, dear." She looks at me as if to say, "Who?" She does not recognize *dear*. Wanting to move from destination A to B, I say, "Come on, boo." This time she chastises me by giving me "the look" she used to give me years ago when I called her that and she was verbal, although slowly losing her ability to speak. She would say, "I'm not boo!" taking the word literally, and I would retort, "But you're my boo, boo!" Just like now, she gives me that smile that I will do anything to see. The solution is always to just stop and give her a moment and resume walking. We continue on to the recliner and she has picked up her pace, which I'm singing "Hallelujah" for.

Narrative refers to a lived experience as a caregiver with known or unknown meaning. *Critical narrative* refers to a complexity of the lived experiences that, through analysis, allows a voice for positioning in spaces and places in conflict or provides an alternative view in prevailing accepted thought. *Critical disability* theory exploring dis/ability critical race theory notions of disability and ableism that cancel out each other in an effort to appear normal, thereby creating a voice vacuum. Along with this voice vacuum is the historical genetic and social status bindings (Annamma et al., 2018). *Epistemological* suppositions refer to knowledge gained from experiences that may be individually experienced or shared.

Stairs provide a function in life. They represent, objectively, unchanging structuralism that is "symbolic" (Denzin, 2013, p. 130) of barriers faced by individuals with disabilities. This is particularly the case of someone who experiences dementia. As my wife's condition has progressed, deterioration of performance over time becomes more evident every day. To accommodate her basic needs and facilitate her activities of daily living, I assume the role of primary caregiver, along with my daughter as caregiver. Hence, increased attention to her needs is necessary in these areas, in general, and facilitating her descent to the first floor of our home and her ascent to our second floor, in particular.

Stairs evolved from climbing poles, ladders, and footpaths made by humans (Templer, 1992). Essentially, these allowed humans to move up and down levels of terrain or inside of structures. When created, they were made from rocks and roots that allowed people to traverse uneven land. As these paths needed to be more permanent, protected from nature, humans began to solidify the structures with wood and other less erosive substances. Inside, stairs allow spaces to efficiently be organized for maximum use, giving access to internal levels in structures.

When we bought our current home, my wife could run up the first set of eight stairs, turn 180°, and ascend the remaining eight stairs. I estimate it took her no more than 18 seconds to get up the stairs. And while my wife usually took one stair at a time, I distinctly remember her taking multiple steps at a time when she reacted to one of our children talking back. Steps were no barrier to her mothering. Even after my wife was diagnosed with frontal temporal dementia, she still maneuvered the stairs quickly. But as her condition progressed, her ability to negotiate up and down the stairs has sharply diminished on bad days to as much as 30 minutes to get up the stairs.

Stairs can be functionally and aesthetically pleasing but can also pose risk for individuals who experience impaired gait, confused cognition, and perfidy because of compromised depth perception. My wife's perception of the steps of the stairs, as she descends, is made more difficult because she has trouble discerning the end of each step because the wood is the same color. As indicated in the transcription in Table 5.1, repeated and multiple directions are necessary for her to "step down." This is not only related to her memory, which is also an issue, but it is related to her primitive sense of feeling safe and secure. While she perceives the edge of each step, she is unsure of what to do. Constant assurance of the safe space is provided so that she trusts my direction to step down. This is augmented by holding onto the banister on the left and the top newel on the right. In spite of the dementia induced anxiety, she is able to step down with her dominant right foot. Sometimes the confusion impairs her ability to know what to do. When this happens, I ask her if I can help her. Specifically, I ask her if I can move her foot. With her permission, I lift her right foot and place it on the next step down, bend her left knee, while insuring she feels secure by asking, "Are you OK?" or "Are you alright?" She will usually respond by saying, "Yes," or nodding affirmatively. Once secure, I help her bring her left foot to the same step as her right foot. Once both feet are aligned on the lower step, I check with her to ensure she feels safe before initiating the next step down. Before the next step, to reduce anxiety and guide her to the next step down, I move her dominant right hand down on the wall and her left hand down on the railing. Over time, we learned the importance of moving her left and right hands slightly down to help her anticipate the next step. Our understanding of the placement of her hands has helped us efficiently assist my wife move up and down the stairs. Each step down requires simultaneous actions from the step above until we reach the bottom floor. Our home is the only place we have to navigate stairs, as other places have elevators or, when we visit other people's homes, we remain on their first floor.

Stairs and Continence Issues

Going downstairs is a typical daily activity on good days. Intense confusion marks her bad days. This is usually gauged by her fluency of movement and level of confusion. Her ease of walking as she gets out of bed and moves to different rooms upstairs helps us discern good and bad days. These days are not easily differentiated. An aspect of this probe has to do with my wife's continence issues. This aspect permeates much of her daily quality of life because of confusion. As caregiver, I have come to understand the magnitude of excrement not only in maneuvering stairs but also in moving through the day. This is because of the confusion associated with these daily bodily functions. Normal excrement function occurs with ease by going to the bathroom for the activity and related behaviors such as subsequent cleaning. In contrast and depending on the dementia level, a person may experience confusion about the sensation and what to do about it. In my wife's case, at the moderate level, the sensation and need to excrete are confused with when to, even in the bathroom. And even when she does relieve herself, she often feels that her bladder is still full. The confusion is more evident in my observation of her fecal retention for multiple related reasons. One reason is because of privacy issues that are connected to when to defecate. In noticeable instances, she will not if I am in the bathroom with her. My daughter and my wife's attendant have not concurred with my experience in this respect. Even alone, however, she may not use the bathroom because of this confusion. When this is the case, multiple issues converge. Because she is confused and tightly holding everything in, walking becomes not only painful for her but also significantly incapacitates her, thereby restricting movement. When she is able to use the bathroom, facilitating her walking around the house, navigating up and down stairs occurs with relative ease. In comparison, negotiating the stairs to the first floor becomes labored with my wife attempting to control bodily functions. When I realize this effort, I ask her, "Does it hurt?" When she replies affirmatively, I tell her that we should hurry downstairs so she can go to the bathroom. Interestingly, she makes an effort to move down the stairs. But, descending the stairs, although more intentional now on her part, is still a slow process. My wife's ability to navigate the stairs in our house intersects with the progression of dementia that has diminished her cognitive ability across all of her activities of daily living (see Table 2.1, Chapter 2). As a result, I assumed the role of caregiver. This includes, but is not limited to, getting in and out of bed, grooming and dressing, and feeding my wife.

Table 5.1. Recording (Selected)—Descending Stairs

Caregiver (C): Are you ready to go downstairs?

Wife (W): Mmm-hmm [meaning "yes"].

C: OK, let's stand up and walk to the stairs.

Helping her stand up from recliner.

Lead her from recliner in bedroom to game room to top of stairs.

Maneuver her to put right hand on top newel and left hand on wall railing of stairs.

Line both feet in front of the thread nosing

At top of stairs

Step 1

C: Let's Step down, Mommy. Repeat, Step down, Repeat May I help you?

W: Yes.

C: Can I lift your foot? *Lifts right foot and places on next step.*

W: *Steps down.*

Step 2

C: *Gently guides her with hand to bend her knee while spotting her as she steps to the lower stair.*
Step down, Mommy.

C: Good. Let's move your hand right here.

C: *Moves her right hand to a stair spindle and left hand lower on the railing.*

C-OK, step down. Repeat, Repeat

W: *Steps down.*

C: *Helps bring down left foot with right foot.*

Step down, Repeat, Repeat.

Steps down with right foot. Bend leg at her knee and she brings the other foot down. Does it hurt? Does it hurt? Repeated

Step 3

C: Step down. Step down.
Step down. Repeated. Repeated
Step down. Step down, Mommy.
Come on, put your foot down.
Step down. Step down.
Step down. Step down.
Step down again.
Step down. Step down.

Step 4

C: Step down. And let's put your hand right here.
Yes, yes. Step down.
Step down.
Step down, Mommy.
Come on, step down.
Step down.
Step down.

Step 5

C: You alright? You alright? You okay?

SAFELY AND SOFTLY UP AND DOWN THE STAIRCASE

OK good.

W: Un-hum.

C: You alright.
Come on. Come on.
And put your hand right there, okay.
Let's step down.

Step 6

C: Come on.
Put your foot down.
Put your foot down. Put your foot down, Mommy.
Come on. Step down.
Come on, Mommy, so I can get your lunch. Are you ready to eat?

W: Eat?

C-Yeah, you want to eat?
Come on, put your foot down.
Step down.
Step down, Mommy.
Put your hand up here step down.

Step 7

C: You put your hand right here.
Come on step down. Mommy, put your foot down.
Thank you, baby step down again.
Step down. Step down.
Step down. Step down. Step down.
Step down Mommy.
Mommy step down, down.
Step down mommy. Come on.
Step down. Step down mommy. There you go. OK. Are you alright.

Step 8

C: Can you step down again?
Step down again. Step down.
Step down mom.
Step down, Mommy.
You OK?
You alright?
Step down, Mommy. Come on, step down. Step down, Mommy.

W: I want to step down.

C: Good! Step down. Come on.
Step down.
Step down.
Come on, put your foot down.
Step down. Step down. Step down.
Step down. Step down, Mommy.
Good job.

[*I sigh.*]

Step 9—Landing.

We walk around to next set of eight stairs.

Arriving Downstairs

"What is all of this?" my wife shrieked when I led her downstairs one morning when she could still speak. It was a statement, made in a tone from her former self, not for dialog or discussion. It had that tinge of infrequent judgment and combativeness that made me look at her with a past expectation that reminded me not to take the bait because she was setting me up to react. Over the course of our marriage, I'd learned to avoid this premeditated trigger. Premeditated because she planned to make her point early to get it over with in the morning or so that it would be done with before we went to bed. This was surreal because for a moment, I had my old wife back. My response was to ask her if she had something on her mind. Today, like she did in the past, she sighed and said, "Yes." I was waiting for her to tell me what she meant. But she just laughed, which was a pleasing response for me because of her radiant smile. She was surprised to see the mound of laundry to be folded, not to mention that the room was in disarray. But it had been the same the night before; she just didn't remember. I could tell she wanted to fold the mound of clothes, towels, and bedding I had thrown on a chair and ottoman in the far corner of our living room, or den as my wife called it. In the house I grew up in, it would be the "back room" because it is in the back of the house. In our house, the front room is my wife's formal living room with her formal white sofas and wood furniture. She had strong feelings about having these rarely used formal entertaining spaces. In the formal living room are unique antique and antique-ish furniture and paintings my wife personally picked to augment the room. Knowing her mother, I could see similarities, although, on our part, on a less grand scale. The most important piece I contributed to this room is a beautiful oil painting of my wife in her wedding dress I commissioned Tony Sherman to paint a few years after we were married as an anniversary gift. While my wife was embarrassed when I gave it to her, I remember her gazing at the painting and commenting on the beautiful colors the artist painted but never acknowledging her own beauty. In terms of material possessions, it is one of my most prized assets.

Our day is spent watching the news on the TV while at the same time listening to several genres of music. A speaker is placed near her so she can hear the music. Soon after my wife was diagnosed, I learned about the value of music to relieve agitation and anxiety in individuals who experience dementia. Much of the research I read, however, suggested instrumental or classical music. But these genres did not stimulate and calm her as much as her favorite types. Listening to music is a pastime for my wife. Except for prayer, I cannot think of anything more constant in her life than listening to her favorite music. While she appreciated all kinds of music, her all-time favorite genre is soul, with rap, hip-hop, and pop coming in second depending on the hit at the time. In addition to almost any soul music, my wife loved Tupac Shakur and Michael Jackson. She brought into our marriage a box of soul albums. She had albums by Curtis Mayfield, Stevie Wonder, Otis Redding, almost everything made by the Temptations, Smokey Robinson's "The Tracks of My Tears," Marvin Gaye's "I Heard It Through the Grapevine," Aretha Franklin's "You Make Me Feel Like a Natural Woman," and many more. And she sang along whenever she played the songs. Even though the box was a plain cardboard box, its shape seemed to have been made just for albums. While I never counted them, I estimate it was the home to 50 to 60 albums. Tupac and Jackson were initially played from an audiotape, later from CDs, and now from digital formats. While we had an 8-track player and cartridges, these became obsolete after we were married. For some time, we relied on music playlists from our cell phones to play much of my wife's favorite music. Today, we maintain these playlists on the Amazon Echo and, with ease, have Alexa to play anything.

Downstairs, part of our evening routine involves warming up my wife's dinner. I have gotten into the habit of prepping her food on weekends. From the freezer, I remove a rotisserie thigh or breast I've bought cooked, frozen mixed vegetables, and frozen prepped mini potatoes I roasted. After I defrost these, I arrange these on a dish that separates protein, vegetables, and starches; then I microwave her dinner and serve it to her. I cut her chicken into small parts because she can no longer cut it up herself. Because she is unable to use silverware, the small cuts allowed her to pick up the food with her hands and to eat it. Now, however, we feed it to her because she does not see all the food on her plate. We became aware of this when she ate half of her food, implying to us that she may have only seen half of her plate. Eventually, she began to reach for her food, and we would put her hand on her plate. For a while, she seemed to find the finger foods, but later, she seemed not to remember where the food was or could not find it. Trying to grasp the finger foods seemed frustrating to her, and she would stop trying to find them. Because she can no longer swallow her medicine whole, I crush it, mix it in with yogurt, and feed it to her. After we eat dinner, we head upstairs for the evening.

I prefer to tidy up the kitchen before we go upstairs. It has become increasingly irritating to come down in the morning and have to clean the kitchen. But I recognize now that not cleaning in the evening has to do more with the time it takes to help my wife up the stairs, assist her in the bathroom and get into bed, say prayers, and comfort her into calming down to ease her to sleep. As we began to prepare to move upstairs to our bedroom, I hurriedly turned lights out in the bathroom, kitchen, and living room; drew the front curtains closed; and set the alarm. I quickly looked in the kitchen to see how much I would need to clean up in the morning. Unlike my wife, I tend to tidy the kitchen in the morning, using this as devotional time. I reflect on how my wife would not go to bed until she had completely cleaned the kitchen and tidied the house. This was one of her reflection and solitude times of the day, and she guarded this time by encouraging us to leave her space and go to our respective bedrooms. Now our routines had changed, and when possible, I preferred to clean and tidy up downstairs, if possible, before we go upstairs. But if I don't get to it at night, I've learned to give myself permission to get to it when I can and feel good about it.

Easing my wife into sleep takes about 3 to 4 hours from the time she gets into bed. Most evenings, my wife seems to want to get into bed but not go to sleep. Even in total darkness, she may lie in bed with her eyes open until about 10 or 11 p.m.

Climbing the stairs to our bedroom can be more problematic than usual some days. On easy days, we climb the stairs in 3 to 4 minutes. However, more commonly, we climb them in 5 to 10 minutes. On bad days, it may take us as long as 30 minutes to get to the top of the stairs. As I stated earlier, removing bathroom issues ensures that we climb the stairs quickly. On one particular day, my wife was more listless than usual. We'd stayed downstairs later than usual (7:00 p.m.), and she appeared to be tired. When she is like this, she has a harder time climbing the stairs. And, the later we wait, the more challenging climbing the stairs is for her. We moved to the bottom of the stairs in the living room. At the bottom of the stairs, I repeatedly coached my wife to step up. It took us approximately 20 minutes from bottom to top, with a lot of coaching such as "Lift your leg," "Lift your foot," or "Step up." Processing commands takes her some time. And the same command may or may not elicit the expected outcome as it did previously. Memory, of course, is another issue, thereby making prediction problematic. The command "lift your foot" might work one day and not the next. Or it might work for one step and not the next. Although consistency is important with my wife, the same command does not always register. Advancing her right hand up the railing while holding on to her left hand helps guide her up the stairs. Ideally, she steps up on her own, but on some occasions, when it is taking her a long time to process, if I gain her permission to lift her foot up to the next step, she will begin to step up on her own for several steps or until we reach the top of the stairs.

Over time I grew to understand that my tone, precise language, and lag time were important. Speaking in a soft, warm tone, in almost a whisper, helped facilitate my wife following instructions to climb the stairs. Also of importance were the amount and the succinctness of the language I used. I always knew that time for processing was important. However, I was often surprised when my wife stepped up or down during quiet moments on the stairs. She was "just" acting on the last processed prompt I may have given her a minute before. This reminded me to be patient.

Axiological Underpinnings

Axiology refers to the constant relational value positionality I experience in the care for my wife. I espouse that axiological consciousness, like the permanent and functional stairs mentioned earlier, is a strong and positive caregiver value that precludes other important displaced values. This is evident in my husband role changing to the new role of caregiver/husband. Caregiving has become my most important role in my relationship with my wife while not weakening the importance of my husband role. After my wife's diagnosis, new legal and medical guardian roles were necessary and created, thereby adding an even more morally conscious role of guardian. My new role became caregiver, husband, legal guardian, and medical guardian. As my wife's husband, I did not possess the authority to manage her affairs. Our bequeathing all possessions and holdings to each other upon either one's death did not grant legal or medical guardianship. Legal actions to create licit documents were required to manage not only her medical but also her financial affairs.

As with the stairs, my caregiver/husband role is not flexible in terms of my commitment and responsibility to my wife. Alongside axiology, ontological *suppositions* refer to complex lived realities and their meanings about dementia in a valued person. In caregiving autoethnography, the caregiver participates in the known and is evidenced in the experience with the person receiving the care (Heron, 1996). Collectively, axiology and ontology exist as philosophical bearings, serving as foundations for explaining the phenomenon of caregiving, or why I do it. But to understand the collective phenomenon, separating them for the purpose of exploration is helpful.

As I consider axiology, rhetorical (to think about) or literal (when action is taken) questions that arise include What are my ethics, morals, or values about caregiving? and How are the ethics in this chapter different from those in Chapter 2? I am mindful that for the purposes of my autoethnographic exploration of caregiving, ethics, morals, and values are synonymous. How did I come to know good or bad? The most important questions might be, How do my values affect me and my caregiving? How do I know I have values? and To what extent do my values guide me to make moral decisions? Human growth and development studies suggest that we are not born with moral awareness, but with cognitive development and as our brain evolves during early childhood (Kohberg, 1976), our values consciousness emerges and matures throughout our life span. They evolve from complex experiences of sensing what feels good and bad from our parents', community's, and society's interpretation and shaping of what is right and wrong. When I violated known or unknown values, what thinking brought me to moral behavior?

Ethics or morality can be traced back to the ancient African philosopher Ptahhotep (ca. 2414 BCE), who is considered to be the "first ethical philosopher" (Adu-Asamoa, 2008, p. 23). Ptahhotep encouraged man's accord with nature. He further gave instructions on living through his writings in *The Teachings of Ptahhotep: The Oldest Book in the World* (Ptahhotep, 1909/2016). The book is formatted with an introduction and conclusion and 37 maxims of wisdom from ancient times (Gerlach, 2020). Ptahhotep espoused wisdom around "moderation, kindness, justice and honesty." These instructions (Fontaine, 1981) on morality include limericks on topics such as the evil of old age, the value of education, how to win an argument, table manners at court, advice to a family man, and good conduct (Fontaine, 1981, pp. 58–59). Other instructions focus on ethics of argument, manners for guests, fathers, just judging, treatment of servants, duties of the great, friendship, obedience, and generational relationships (Ptahhotep, 1909/2016, pp. 41–61).

Although debated but credited with ideals of ethics, Plato (428–348 BCE), and Aristotle (385–322 BCE) studied in Africa and later returned to Greece. Their study in Egypt had a great influence on their later thought on the subject of ethics. Plato, a student of Socrates and Aristotle's teacher, is best known for his (1906) book *Republic*. In it, Plato engages in a Socratic dialog about the abstract good in the world and in the individual.

Aristotle, after Alexander the Great's pillage of Egyptian libraries, took their holdings and promoted them as his own (Adu-Asamoa, 2008). With this foundational and philosophical knowledge, Aristotle forged ideals of African morality into the Greek experience and its larger society of the time (Gyekye, 2011). Aristotle's theses include what have become ideals on "character . . . happiness . . . flourishing, virtue, excellence, pleasure and the proper relationship between human beings and the divine" (Kraut, 2018, p. 2).

Historically across African languages, ethics or morality have been translated to mean good, bad, or evil "character," as observed in ancient Africa and Greece (Gyekye, 2011; Kraut, 2018). In modern and postmodern societies, while African ethics has a broader meaning, the concept of "character of the individual matters most in . . . moral life and thought" (Gyekye, 2011, p. 4). Character is attained through African cultural assimilation as a result of being. An African "maxim" of the Akan of southern Ghana is "one is not born with a bad 'head,' but one takes it on from the earth." African cultural philosophy is expected to instill an epistemology of a learned moral lifestyle that is specific and taught by everyday interactions with others and nature. As a result of good moral "habits" (Gyekye, 2011, p. 5), character is developed to reflect who the person is.

In addition to character, other axiological ethical or moral consciousness has been constructed by Gyekye (2011) as collective[1] African principles that include moral personhood (moral state of being or existing), brotherhood, the common good, social responsibility, and duty. Moral personhood

---

1 Representing Ghana, Nigeria, Yoruba, Lovedu (northern South Africa), and Nyakyusa (formerly German East Africa).

to another or other people is a value in African people. An unraveling of this idea can be compartmentalized into understandings of what it means to be a person in the human race compared to lacking personhood but of the human race. The former is the desired status and the latter is the undesirable status. To be told that one is not a person is an insult. Behaviors judged to be attributed to individuals as "not a person" include "cruel, wicked, selfish, ungenerous or unsympathetic" (Gyekye, 2011, p. 5). On the other hand, people are not assumed to be born with prosocial behaviors but that these are instilled as a result of metaphysical moral interactions with nature and people. For example, it is a desire to be a steward of nature by only using what is needed to live. Personhood ascribes to "norms" of being of "good character," being "generous," "peaceful," "humble," and having "respect for others" (Gyekye, 2011, p. 6). Along with personhood is the "wherewithal," or character, to choose between "good and evil."

Within religion is positioned a sense of "humanity" that provides vital structures saturating African moral life. These structures set lifestyles that are dichotomized into "good or bad" and "right or wrong" (Gyekye, 2011, p. 7) and direct all moral behaviors. African philosophy draws moral guidance from not only religion but also from the concepts of the good of humankind that "builds up society" (McVeigh, 1974, p. 9, as cited in Gyekye, 2011), "upholds the social structure" (Drige & Krige, 1954, p. 9, as cited in Gyekye, 2011), and achieves the "greatest happiness and good" that results in "utilitarian ... altruism" (Molema, 1920, p. 9, as cited in Gyekye, 2011).

The African trait of regard for "others" over the self is intertwined with the concept of "brotherhood." It is a gender-neutral concept extolling compassion, self-denial, consideration, and care; even if individuals do not have personhood status, they are treated as brothers because they are human beings. Brotherhood extends "hospitality, generosity, concern for others and communal feeling" (Gyekye, 2011, p. 11). The phenomenon of brotherhood is a moral designation and extends beyond kindship. Gyekye (2011) explains that brotherhood has no boundaries and transcends "human biology, race,[2] ethnicity, or culture" (p. 11). It does not have familial boundaries.

---

2 Gyekye (2011) states that the word *race* does not have an "autochthonous African language" equivalent except for languages that include derivatives from languages such as Arabic.

Tantamount to humanity and brotherhood in African philosophy are the ideals of "common good" (Gyekye, 2011, p. 12) and communal responsibility. In meeting the common good of the community, individual needs are met. The societal institutions of law, politics, and the economy function in accord to achieve "peace, happiness or satisfaction (human flourishing), justice, dignity respect and so on" (Gyekye, 2011, p. 12) to inoculate society for purely individual pursuits that do not benefit the whole and thereby achieving a "social morality" (p. 13). Furthermore, successful individual pursuits require communal support that are "socially, economically, emotionally, and psychologically" (Gyekye, 2011, p. 13) reciprocally aided by society.

Finally, Gyekye (2011) explains the demands of "duty" (p. 15) on citizens of African culture. Duty, as a culmination of the aforementioned African mores—character, personhood, brotherhood, humanity, and the common good—along with humanity, serves as the foundation for its axiology. These duty mores beginning at home extend to the milieu, then to the country, and then to the world.

My sense of duty to my wife may be explained using these African mores. In reflecting on how my cumulative mores were intentionally taught to me, specific teachings come to mind. I can remember my parents building character through routines, such as completing chores, church, and the Boy Scouts, under their watchful eyes at home and through many other involvements and affiliations. Within character, my parents sought to build a sense of personhood in an effort to instill who we were while developing a sense of right and wrong. I recall my mother stressing appropriate behavior at school over achieving perfect grades. As I reflected on this many years later, I could see her concern that her Black boys not become part of the criminal justice system. This could have been easy to accomplish given society's trend. In building our personhoods, when I did get in trouble with teachers and in the community, my parents knew if the reported behavior was indicative of who they knew me to be.

Brotherhood, in a narrow sense, was important to my father because he told us that we were fortunate to have siblings because he grew up as a single child. He would go on to talk about not having brothers and sisters and how this made him feel lonely. He would tell us this whenever we fought. In the broader sense, my dad stressed making good friendships based on mutual respect and understanding. He would often ask us how others might feel about a life situation we saw them experiencing. Connected to brotherhood was my parents' instilling a sense of humanity in their children. During the summer when my mother was not teaching, I remember her gathering us together with several neighborhood boys to teach us manners. Not being open to it, we asked her why we needed to learn to open the door for ladies, help old ladies across the street, pull a chair out for ladies, or eat with the right utensil. Each summer, her answers were the same with a rationale and with the assertion of her authority by saying, "Because I want you to know . . ." Those were the words we learned not to challenge. In addition to concern for humanity were instructions such as to leave our surrounding better than we found them. By this my mother might be talking about putting loose paper or a can in the park or elsewhere in the garbage. It seems like we were always told by our parents and at church to not waste food, water, or electricity because we were expected to be stewards of the earth. This included altruistic giving at church and the broader world community.

I say all this about axiological or moral grounding to articulate my sense of duty to my wife. It is more than just my wedding vows, which are important; I seek meaning for my spiritual embodiment pulling toward an ethical ethos. From a critical perspective and contrary to what some researchers (Bergman & Pulling, 2020; Chen & Olson, 2015; Cohen, 2012; Hildebrand, 2016; Li et al., 2018; Lindenberger & Meier, 2013; Schulz, 2001; Thimsen, 2020; Valois & Galvin, 2014; Waldrop & Kutner, 2013) of dementia and other disorders suggest feeling "burdened" with caregiving, African ethics reject this notion (Gyekye, 2011). Instead, an "ethic of duty" (Gyekye, 2011, p. 15) that draws from cumulative instilled embodiments of moral development across the life span is mandatory of individuals. African culture does not deny the realities of caregivers, which include physical and emotional fatigue, depression, sleep deprivation, frustration and feelings of inadequacies, and other actualities. It does not ignore the importance of respite and attention to personal well-being. But African philosophy does not accept that duty is an optional "right" (Gyekye, 2011, p. 15). Instead, duty is based on a "consciousness of needs rather than rights" (Gyekye, 2011, p. 15). More specifically, this concept expects the caregiver to go "beyond the call of duty" (p. 15) and rejects the ideal of "supererogation" (Gyekye, 2011, p. 15).

Axiological Duty and Supererogation in Comparative Cultures

African philosophy compels its citizens to possess an internalized duty to each other even if the person being cared for suffers long in comparison to the ideal of supererogatory duty in Western culture. Gyekye (2011) points out that the concept of supererogation in Western culture offers the option of excusing caregiving if it is burdensome without condemnation. It would not go against the Western mores and is forgiven in the culture. The ideal of supererogation views performing care as commendable but not obligatory. Moreover, supererogation in Western culture allows a person in need to be consciously abandoned. In fact, while initially noble, in the United States, the course for this practice was legalized in the Community Mental Health Act of 1963,[3] also known as the Deinstitutionalization Act of 1963, under President John F. Kennedy. President Kennedy displayed a genuine sense of duty as he interacted with his sister, who experienced a disability. As an expression of this brotherly devotion, he demonstrated a belief that the quality of life of individuals with disabilities might be improved if they were served in communities rather than experience "custodial isolation" in institutions, thereby "[restoring] them to a useful life" (Papers of John F. Kennedy, 1963, p. 1). The act displayed a national sense of ethical duty toward individuals institutionalized in the United States, even if duty could not be guaranteed as envisioned. President Jimmy Carter passed the Mental Health Systems Act of 1980 to maintain and enhance the efforts of the Kennedy initiative. Unfortunately, within months and with the election of President Ronald Reagan, the Omnibus Budget Reconciliation Act of 1980 repealed President Carter's Mental Health Systems Act. As a consequence of this repeal, long-lasting effects resulted in the broad release of individuals with mental illness from state hospitals who ended up in prison and on the streets. These newly homeless individuals with mental illnesses were expected to medicate themselves, navigate social services for mental health care, and secure work and housing (Torrey, 2014). Ultimately, deinstitutionalization resulted in not only increased prison rates, homelessness, and mental illness but also further objectification (Foucault, 1987) of the most vulnerable people in the United States. Furthermore, the United States excused and codified the ideal of

---

3 Also known as the Mental Health Act of 1963.

supererogationism nationally. One might wonder how people can grow up in the same country but possess very different ideas of moral duty.

Moral duty in any society begins with instilled values and is required for professional caregivers in exchange for payment with the assumption that services are delivered by a person with such embodied character. The moral duty voluntary or informal caregivers provide is based on trust and equal to that expected from a professional caregiver. Knowing the value any caregiver places on a person's life is important. My wife and I have been blessed with professional and nonprofessional caregivers and friends who are thoughtful, attentive, and impactful. Of course, visiting friends and family who are in nursing homes or "shut in" demonstrates a value taught to me from an early age, as my parents taught us this starting very young. This value was further developed as community service by high school and college teachers as we visited with elderly residents in nursing homes and in the homes of teachers. It is the professional caregiver (a stranger to us) who enters my wife's space and immediately places a throw blanket on my wife because of the *cutis anserine*, or "goosebumps," she sees on my wife's arms, something I have not picked up on while sitting beside her, or the doctor who, when she opens the door and walks into the room, begins by talking directly to my wife (a common behavior of hers) and touches her while noticing that my wife did not respond to her as she came in. While examining her, she points out to me that my wife has a buildup of earwax and prescribes a way to remove it. Another example is the occupational therapist who spent extra time with her patient (a family member) marking crossword puzzles because the patient could not move her arms or write. And a final example of the demonstration of the moral duty of a Registered Nurse working in a nursing home who tells the family of a patient (family member) to bring artifacts from home to make the room more familiar to the patient and follows up on her recommendation. Other examples exist, too many to list, of the sense of moral duty of professional and nonprofessionals caregivers whose practice and lives have intersected with the lives of my wife and me.

Sadly, since my wife's dementia diagnosis, I am more cognizant of unethical, morally deficient, and supererogational care shown to her and others with neurological disorders. Although these experiences are few, they have been eidetic memories and heartbreaking. I have observed mostly professional caregivers, including medical professionals, who, attending with my wife, treat those affected with neurological disorders as objects, not as valued human beings. Examples of this include seeing a naked person (stranger) in a nursing home hallway while visiting a family member or a person (a friend and family member) who has not been attended to in a nursing home or private residence for hours. But most surprising to me are personal experiences of doctors who, when they came into the examination rooms, did not look at either my wife or me and did not speak or touch my wife during her entire visit while making a diagnosis. Another doctor when entering the exam room asked, "Who am I seeing today?" Obviously, this question sent up red flags about the attention he paid to my wife's chart and to her. This reminded me of my son's pediatrician, who would come into the room, looked at him, and ask the same question (as he often did jokingly to my children), to which my son would wittingly point to me. Matching his wit, the doctor asked him to list my symptoms. This was not the case with the physician attending my wife on this visit. He did not know who he was seeing that day. The most egregious abuse I observed, however, was recorded using a spy-type camera and released through the media by a family of a person experiencing dementia and a professional caregiver violently hitting and yelling at the lady as punishment for something she had done. When the lady tried to get away from the caregiver, she was followed, punched, and yelled at by the caregiver. I wonder how a person could inflict such evil on another person.

While Nicolae Râmbu (2015) indicates such a lack of moral consciousness is an "axiological blindness and tyranny of the values [that] transform the affected person by turning them into an axioclast or, in other words, a destroyer of values" (p. 64), he visits the notion mentioned earlier of supererogation as he addresses the ontology that axiological consciousness may result in not all values being applied with the same passion by man. But he cautions that "adequate coverage of some values fatally means ignoring others" (Râmbu, 2015, p. 64). Râmbu also indicates that values do not occur in a vacuum and are not "indifferent" (2015, p. 68). Rather, moral consciousness occurs in context and is always available to us. Thus, quality caregiving, as discerned in the earlier examples, is subjective because of our free will but dependent on moral duty. Râmbu insists that when "man does not master the value, but the value masters him" (2015, p. 68), value tyranny occurs. This tyranny becomes a power that is misguided and mistaken for noble value. In terms of self-reflection of my values, using Râmbu's concept of mastering them, with caregiving at the core to ensure that my wife's needs are fully met, I must constantly examine my behavior to ensure that my focus on moral values is multidirectional and balanced. A one-directional value would be, for example, my ignoring my wife's needs until a professional attendant arrived because it is what the attendant is paid to do or deciding that only women can bathe my wife and deny her a bath because I am a man. While all caregivers should be held accountable for providing quality care, these are examples of false and single-minded caregiver values. Furthermore, being inconsiderate of professional and involuntary caregivers is also one-directional and is devoid of value consciousness. For example, as I arrange care for my wife, is it appropriate for me to abuse outside caregivers? Should I expect them to provide care I would not provide? If one of the duties of the hired caregiver is to cook and clean for my wife, should I expect the person to cook and clean for me? Does relying on others to care for my wife cause a detachment in the relationship with my wife? Could quality care for my wife be delivered in a nursing home or care facility?

Conclusion

> *The Lord is my light and my salvation; whom shall I fear? the Lord is the strength of my life; of whom shall I be afraid?*
>
> *When the wicked, even mine enemies and my foes, came upon me to eat up my flesh, they stumbled and fell.*
>
> *Though a host should encamp against me, my heart shall not fear: though war should rise against me, in this will I be confident.*
>
> *One thing have I desired of the Lord, that will I seek after; that I may dwell in the house of the Lord all the days of my life, to behold the beauty of the Lord, and to enquire in his temple.*
>
> PSALMS 27:1–4 KJV

As I bring this construction of autoethnography mixed with phenomenology to an end, I am humbled at the amount of theory, philosophy, and practice from the rich scholarship in the field. The heart of autoethnography is found in the phenomenological souls of the collective subjective stories of the main and significant other characters. Drawing on reflections of memory pieces and journal entries, a collective emerged in this academic book. Whereas the academic exploration of theory and philosophy in autoethnography and phenomenology is intellectually instructive, the reflective journey through them during the season of husband caregiving is edifying self-work. Constructing my autoethnography afforded me the opportunity to reflect on personal experiences with caring for the most important person in my life as she lives through dementia and to search through established theories, speculating on new theories, philosophies, and phenomenologies. Personally, the journey has started the process of disrupting my emotional impasse and moving through the shock of my trauma and ongoing burden of watching the love of my life dwindle daily. My journey to and through autoethnography has presented me the opportunity to read and learn, write and learn, and reflect and learn about the constant interceptions of theories and their applications to life. This grand exercise was very gratifying.

There are many more relevant theories and philosophies I wish I could have explored along with personal discourse. The theory I was able to touch on provided a springboard for future study and autoethnographic writings. Reflecting on the topics I explored allowed me to venture beyond the edges of where I had previously only temporally explored, laying bare the vulnerabilities broached in these pages or those addressed later. To some extent, journeying through autoethnographic narrative was uncomfortable because of the junctures along the way. These junctures were often familiar places but not deeply explored for reasons of time, sensitivity, or process. My disclosure allowed for the revelation of vulnerability tensions in my life with possible transformations. Although the change does not come with a road map, the examined experiences prepare for the future.

My son taking his life is an example of a topic I broached but controlled the discourse on because of the complexity of profound grief, compounded loss, faith issues, and the impact it has on his mother, his sister, and me. Because I do not feel ready to engage in the deep and emotional reflection needed to explore this issue, I am deferring it and considering the phenomenon in future writing. Exploring relational spaces helped me reflect on the meanings for those closest to me. Addressing the emptiness his death left and the subsequent bereavement is an area I feel compelled to address in a separate discourse for not only the reasons stated earlier but others not disclosed as well. Continued therapeutic support is a component of this future endeavor. And while autoethnography could extend discourse and therapeutic options, I would like to look at other alternatives. A generic qualitative inquiry is what I've started, with the intention of selecting a single or even a mixed-method approach.

Reflecting on my disclosed collective narrative brings to mind thoughts of gratification that I am able to care for my wife with the help of our daughter and other trusted people. As I reflect on this discourse, I can't help but feel what I have shared is corny, aggrandizing, and trite. But I am pleased to have explored autoethnography from the perspective of caregiving.

In these reflections are realities or ontological bearings. Just as I would do many things over in life and wish many things were different, those things, good or bad, are the experiences that bring me to a point in my life of appreciation for the most important aspect of it, my wife. For a while after my wife's diagnosis, I felt tormented with bargaining thoughts, asking God to afflict me instead of my wife. But, as I processed my thoughts, I realized that my purpose in the here and now was to care for my wife. Every experience in my life prepared me for my role as my wife's caregiver. And I'm good with that!

Reader Thought Questions and Further Reading

1. What is the significance of stairs in the autoethnography?
2. Compare and contrast the structuralism of the stairs to a qualitative change in the caregiving, dementia, and disability narrative.
3. What role does axiology play in a person's life?
4. How might "supererogation" be demonstrated in a person's life?
5. How is supererogationism an oxymoron (Gyekye, 2011)?
6. What are the beginning, middle, and end of this autoethnography?
7. What is the setting in this autoethnography?
8. What is the relationship of the protagonist to other characters?
9. What is the point (or points) of view?

10. What might be the climax of this autoethnography?
11. What are the themes in the story?
12. What style did the author use?

References

Adu-Asamoa, B. (2008, October). Greek philosophers who came to Africa to study. *New African*, (477).

Annamma, S. A., Ferri, B. A., & Connor, D. J. (2018). Disability critical race theory: Exploring the intersectional lineage, emergence, and potential futures of discrit in education. *Review of Research in Education, 42*, 46–71.

Bergman, E. J., & Pulling, B. W. (2020). Chapter 12—caregiving of the older adult. In D. Avers & R. A. Wong (Eds.), *Guccione's geriatric physical therapy* (4th ed., pp. 265–282). Mosby.

Chen, M. L., & Olson, H. C. (2015). Chapter 34—sleep in fetal alcohol spectrum disorders. In R. R. Watson (Ed.), *Modulation of sleep by obesity, diabetes, age, and diet* (pp. 313–319). Academic Press.

Cohen, D. A. (2012). Chapter 52—sleep disorders associated with dementia. In T. J. Barkoukis, J. K. Matheson, R. Ferber, & K. Doghramji (Eds.), *Therapy in sleep medicine* (pp. 656–665). W. B. Saunders.

Denzin, N. K. (2013). Interpretive autoethnography. In S. H. Jones, T. E. Adams, & C. Ellis (Eds.), *Handbook of autoethnography* (p. 130). Routledge.

Fontaine, C. R. (1981). A modern look at ancient wisdom: The instruction of Ptahhotep revisited. *The Bibical Archaeologist, 44*(3), 155–160.

Foucault, M. (1987). *Mental illness and psychology*. Berkeley: University of California Press.

Gerlach, E. (2020, July 21). *Egyptian ethics and philopshy: Hardjedef and Ptahhotep* [Video]. YouTube. https://www.youtube.com/watch?v=ciihKSfiIec

Gyekye, K. (2011, Fall). African ethics. In E. N. Zalta (Ed.), *The Stanford encyclopedia of philosophy*. https://plato.stanford.edu/archives/fall2011/entries/african-ethics/

Heron, J. (1996). *Co-operative inquiry*. Sage.

Heron, J., & Reason, P. (1997). A participatory inquiry paradigm. *Qualitative Inquiry, 3*(3), 274–294. https://link.gale.com/apps/doc/A20608060/ITOF?u=txshracd2540&sid=ITOF&xid=c3a877ae

Hildebrand, M. W. (2016). Chapter 15—caregiving after stroke. In G. Gillen (Ed.), *Stroke rehabilitation* (4th ed., pp. 309–327). Mosby.

Kohberg, L. (1976). Moral stages and moralization: The cognitive development approach. In T. Lickona (Ed.), *Moral development and behavior: Theory, research and social issues* (pp. 31–53). Holt, Rinehart and Winston.

Kraut, R. (2018, Summer). Aristotle's ethics. In E. N. Zalta (Ed.), *Stanford ency-*

clopedia of philosophy. https://plato.stanford.edu/archives/sum2018/entries/aristotle-ethics/

Li, Y., Saini, S., Caine, K., & Connelly, K. (2018). 7—checking-in with my friends: Results from an in-situ deployment of peer-to-peer aging in place technologies. In R. Pak & A. C. McLaughlin (Eds.), *Aging, technology and health* (pp. 147–178). Academic Press.

Lindenberger, E., & Meier, D. E. (2013). Chapter 56—what special considerations are needed for individuals with amyotrophic lateral sclerosis, multiple sclerosis, or Parkinson disease? In N. E. Goldstein & R. S. Morrison (Eds.), *Evidence-based practice in palliative medicine* (pp. 317–329). W. B. Saunders.

National Council on Aging. (2020). *Falls prevention: Keeping older adults safe and active.* https://www.ncoa.org/healthy-aging/falls-prevention/

Papers of John F. Kennedy. (1963). Special message on mental illness and mental retardation. In *Reflecting on JFK's legacy of community-based care: Presendential papers.* President's Office Files. Legislative Files. https://www.samhsa.gov/homelessness-programs-resources/hpr-resources/jfk's-legacy-community-based-care

Plato. (1906). *The republic of Plato* (J. L. Davies & D. J. Vaughan, Trans.). Macmillian.

Ptahhotep. (2016). *The teachings of Ptahhotep: The oldest book in the World* (B. G. Gunn, Trans.). Martino Publishing. (Original work published 1909)

Râmbu, N. (2015). Two axiological illnesses. *Jounal of Human Values, 21*(1), 64–71.

Schulz, R. (2001). Caregiver burden. In N. J. Smelser & P. B. Baltes (Eds.), *International encyclopedia of the social & behavioral sciences* (pp. 1476–1479). Pergamon.

Templer, J. (1992). *The staircase: History and theories.* Massachusetts Institute of Technology. https://books.google.com/books?id=hwnQYdhIHDwC&printsec=frontcover&source=gbs_ge_summary_r&cad=0#v=onepage&q&f=false

Thimsen, K. (2020). 4—interpersonal violence and the elderly. In A. Carney (Ed.), *Elder abuse* (pp. 85–105). Academic Press.

Torrey, E. F. (2014). *American psychosis: How the federal government destroyed the mental health treatment system.* Oxford University Press.

Valois, L., & Galvin, J. E. (2014). The role of the family in the care and management of patients with dementia. In B. Dickerson & A. Atri (Eds.), *Dementia: Comprehensive principles and practice* (pp. 609–621). Oxford University Press.

Waldrop, D., & Kutner, J. S. (2013). Chapter 73—what can be done to improve outcomes for caregivers of patients with serious illness? In N. E. Goldstein & R. S. Morrison (Eds.), *Evidence-based practice in palliative medicine* (pp. 429–435). W. B. Saunders.

Epilogue

I find myself being hypervigilant in caring for my wife, looking for any pain or need she might have. Over time, I have evolved to a less urgent stance. I have realized that I pass on my feeling of urgency or calmness to my wife. I realize much of my issue with this is my feeling that I need to finish dressing, grooming, cooking, and transfer this sense of urgency to my wife, which causes her to feel rushed. I often remind myself to pace feeding my wife so that she has time to chew her food. I understand that part of this is because there is always something else to do after I finish the task at hand. On occasion I noticed that she was moving her body and seemed to be trying to say something I did not understand. I could see her excitement in her eyes, and she began to move her body from side to side in a kind of swaying. I did not know how to interpret her behavior, as I had not seen it before. I could not detect that she was in pain. On the radio played a soulful tune with a familiar refrain that I realized my wife was singing and dancing to. To verify that she was actually singing and dancing, I watched her bob her head, and when the refrain played again, she sang it again. Before the song ended, we sang the refrain together.

Along this journey, I recognize my faith as a constant source of support. Without it, I would not have the strength to endure my struggles and great losses, both present and in the past. I know God has not wanted me to experience any of the pain caused by my losses, but He knew they would happen. Yet He did not cause them and is saddened by them, nor did He prevent them in His divine will. It is a figurative likening to "manna from heaven." Through the experience of my wife experiencing dementia and my son's death, I have gained a deeper awakening in my faith and trust in my Lord and Savior Jesus Christ. God's faithfulness has restored my soul. And even though I have not always been faithful, I have always believed in Him and He has blessed me and never left my side, always making His greatness present. He sustains me and gives me clarity during my confusing fog.

> *I have set the LORD always before me: because he is at my right hand, I shall not be moved.*
>
> PSALMS 16:8, KJV

About the Author

Dr. Donald R. Collins is Professor of Educational Leadership and Counseling in the Whitlowe R. Green College of Education at Prairie View A&M University (PVAMU). He is a board member of the HBCU (Historically Black Colleges and Universities) Faculty Development Network and the Texas National Association for Multicultural Education. He is a coeditor of a special issue of the *Qualitative Inquiry* that focuses on institutionalized racism in qualitative inquiry. Dr. Collins has more than 40 years of professional experience in psychology and education that spans teaching, counseling, assessment, and administration.

Dr. Collins earned his PhD in educational psychology from Texas A&M University. He earned his master's degree in educational psychology from Texas Tech University and his Bachelor of Science in English and history from Lubbock Christian College.

Dr. Collins has published in the areas of qualitative research, higher education accreditation, assessment, and multicultural education. He authored *Conducting Multi-Generational Qualitative Research in Education: An Experiment in Grounded Theory* (Peter Lang). The book outlines a methodology for viewing multiple generations of African Americans, specifically those who were called or called themselves Negro, Colored, Black, or African American (NCBAA). He has also published scholarly articles on qualitative research and higher education assessment and a book chapter (Peter Lang) titled "African American Children: Early Childhood Education—Recollections and Life Stories," in G. S. Cannella and L. D. Soto (Eds.), *Childhoods: A Handbook* (Peter Lang). Dr. Collins has received recognition by the Coalition for Critical Qualitative Inquiry as a "Critical Qualitative Scholar." He was honored by the Texas National Association for Multicultural Education for "Distinguished Service." He was recognized by the American Educational Research Association as a "Scholar of Color." He has also delivered scholarly presentations at the local, state, national and international levels. Dr. Collins has research interests in qualitative research, diversity, student learning, school evaluation, and school improvement.

He has worked in the public, private, and corporate sectors. Dr. Collins has taught at the undergraduate and graduate levels. He holds Texas Teaching and Mid-management certifications. As an educational consultant, Dr. Collins worked with 56 school districts in the Houston area. As an independent consultant, he specializes in program and organizational evaluation, assessment, organizational development, curriculum and instruction, and leadership. He has collaborated with local, state, and national leaders to facilitate regional and district initiatives. Dr. Collins is a member of multiple professional organizations and associations.

Index

A
ABC News, 90
Abilene Christian College, 2
ableism, 105
activities of daily living (ADL), 50, 55–59
Adorno, T., 6
Adu-Asamoa, B., 114, 115
African Americans
    dementia and, 51–52
    insider-outsider status, 42–43
    Also see research
African morality, 115
African mores, 117
Aging, Demographics, and Memory Study (ADAMS), 52, 53
Akan, 115
Alexander the Great, 115
altitude sickness, 90, 91
Alzheimer's Association, 51
Alzheimer's Disease, 61
American Psychiatric Association, 53
Anabo, I.F., 30
Annamma, S.A., 105
ante-predictive life of consciousness, 96
Aristotle, 115
Assal, F., 55
At Home With Grief, 95
Audi, R., 87
autobiography, what forms one, 80–83
autoethnography, 1, 5, 8
    allure of, 34–36
    axiology and, 88–90
    becoming aware of, 8–9
    caregiving and, 80–83
    collaborative, 9
    consent and, 38
    data collection and, 83
    deconstructing, 77
    epistemology and, 87–88
    ethics and, 36
    experiential nature of writing, 83–85
    ineffable eidetic knowings, 96–97
    IRB as ethical practice, 34
    life journaling and, 83
    merging with phenomenology, 11–13
    ontology and, 86
    personal vulnerabilities of author, 37–38
    phenomenological agony and, 92–96
    phenomenology and, 85–92, 103
    somatic anxieties and, 43–45
    triggers and, 37
axiological consciousness, 113–18
axiological suppositions, 8
axiology, 13, 86, 88–90, 103
    duty and, 119–22

B
Bachman, D., 58
Bachman, D.L., 53, 58
Banks, J.A., 42, 43, 45, 81
behavior variant FTD (bvFTD), 51
Belmont Report, 31, 36, 37, 53
Benjamin, W., 6
Bergman, E.J., 118
Black Lives Matter, 97
Blessing of Clarity, 94
Bochner, A., 9, 35
Bohman, J., 6
Boylorn, R.M., 83
brotherhood, 116, 117, 118

C
Cahn-Weiner, D.A., 56
Cameron, S.C., 82
capitalism, 6
care culture, 13
caregiving, 5, 13, 61–62, 62–65, 71–72
    African mores and, 117
    autobiography and, 80–83
    autoethnography and, 81
    axiology and, 113–18
    care for the caregiver, 69–71
    external-insider, 45
    financial cost of, 68–69
    formal and informal, 63
    from caring to, 59
    husband status as, 82–83
    moral duty and, 120
    nutrition and, 67–68
    participatory theory and, 103
    phenomenology and, 85–86
    positive aspects of, 7–8
    sense of duty and, 118
    typical caregiving schedule, 65–66
    values and, 122
    versus caretaking, 62
    Also see journal entries by author
caretaking, 62
Carless, D., 32
Carter, J., 119
Celsus, 29, 30
Chang, H., 81
Chatham-Carpenter, A., 37
Chauvin, D., 97
Chen, M.L., 118
childhood amnesia, 79
Church of Christ (COG), 2, 3
    men's training classes and, 4
Church of God in Christ (COGIC), 1, 2
Code of Hammurabi, 29
Cohen, D.A., 118

collaborative autoethnography, 9
Collins, D.R., 77
Collins, P.H., 42
Columbia University, 6
common good, 117
communal responsibility, 117
Community Mental Health Act of 1963, 119
composite characters, 33
consent, 38–39
Corradetti, C., 6
Creswell, J., 13, 86
critical agony, 92
critical consciousness, 13, 79
critical disability theory, 103, 105
critical inquiry lens, 7
critical narrative, 105
critical qualitative inquiry, 7, 8, 92
critical qualitative methods, 77
critical race theory, 7, 103
Critical Race Theory, 7
critical theory, 6, 103
culture, 82

D
Declaration of Geneva, 30
Declaration of Helsinki, 30
Deinstitutionalization Act of 1963
Delgado, R., 7
dementia, 1
    African Americans and, 51–52
    caregiving and, 50
    causes of, 50–51
    communication issues and, 62
    expenses and, 53
    growth in U.S., 51
    no cure for, 49–50
    relationships and, 59–61
    underreporting of, 52–53
Denzin, N., 9, 105
Diagnostic and Statistical Manual of Mental Disorder (DSM-III-R), 53
Diangelo, R., 7
Dickerson, B., 51, 52
Dillard, C., 94
disability, 105
dis/ability critical race theory, 105
Do Thyself No Harm, 37
Douglas, K., 32
Du Bois, W.E.B., 6, 7
Dunbar, P.L., 38
duty, 117, 118
    axiological, 119–22
    moral, 120

E
Edemekong, P.F., 56
eidetic memories, 120
eidetic reduction, 97
Ellis, C., 9, 35, 77, 81, 94

emancipation from slavery, 6
embodiment, 63
Embree, L., 88
epistemology, 13, 86, 87–88, 103, 105
ethical ethos, 118
ethical mindfulness, 32
ethics, 114, 115
    African Americans as research subjects and, 30
    brief history of, 29–30
    conducting autoethnography and, 36
    consent and, 38–39
    questions about, 32
ethnicity, 82
ethnonursing, 13
experiential learning theory, 85
experiential writing, 83–85

F
Falls Prevention Program, 103
Ferngren, G., 29
Fernandez, A.V., 63
Findlay, J.N., 88
Fisher, J.A., 37
Floyd, G., 97
Fontaine, C.R., 114, 115
formal caregiving, 63
Foucault, M., 119
Francis, M.E., 96
Frankfurt School, 6
Frankl, V., 12
Freire, P., 79
Friesen, P., 53
Fromm, E., 6
frontotemporal dementia (FTD), 1, 10, 50–51
    author's wife's diagnosis of, 55–56
frontotemporal lobar degeneration (FTLD), 51, 61
Frost, R., 84
Fusch, P., 45

G
Galvin, J.E., 62, 63, 68, 118
Gamble, V.N., 37
Gerlach, E., 114
Gey, G.O., 37
Gibbs, A., 80
Giebel, C.M., 57, 63
Glaser, B., 92
Grady, D., 36
Great Migration of Blacks, 17
Gregg, B.H., 12
grief, 93–96
grounded theory, 9, 92
Guba, E.G., 35
Gyekye, K., 8, 115, 116, 118, 119

H
Hamermas, J., 6
Hamrale, A., 68

INDEX

Herlihy, B.J., 95
Harris, A.L., 7
Harris, Y., 30
Hart, H.M., 7
Hart, J.G., 88
Hayes, D.G., 82
HeLa, 37
Hernandez, K.-A.C., 95
Heron, J., 103, 114
Hildebrand, M.W., 118
Hippocratic Oath, 29
Horkheimer, M., 6
Husserl, E., 85

I
I Remember..., 15
idealism, 6
Indigenous-insider knowledge, 45
ineffable, 97
informal caregiving, 63
insider-outsider status, 42–43, 43–45
Institute for Social Research, 6
institutional review board (IRB), 29, 32–34
International Congress of Qualitative Inquiry (ICQI), 8, 9, 92
interpretive analysis, 86

J
Jeffries, S., 6
Jones, S.H., 81
Jonsen, A.R., 30
journal entries by author
    Coffee with my daddy, 24
    Disclosure in Autoethnography, 31–32
    Familial Aspects of Caregiving, 39–42
    Thinking With My Journal, 10–11

K
Kennedy, J.F., 119
Knopman, D.S., 52
Kocet, M.M., 95
Kohberg, L., 114
Kolb, D., 85
Kraut, R., 115
Kutner, J.S., 118

L
Lacks, H., 37
Launer, L.J., 53
Leininger, M., 13
Li, Y., 117
liberal order, 7
Lincoln, Y.S., 35
Lind, C., 77, 79, 80
Lindenberger, E., 118
Lloyd, J., 7
Lowenthal, I.O., 6

M
Maddrell, A., 82, 95, 97
Man's Search for Meaning, 12
Manly, J.J., 53
Mapping Grief, 97
Marcuse, H., 6
Martin, J.N., 83
Marx, K., 7
Marxism, 6
Maternal Connections, 35
Mayeux, R., 53
McAdams, D.P., 7
McFarland, M., 13
McLeod, A.L., 82
meanings, 12–13
Medeiros, K.D., 37
Mehta, K.M., 51, 53
Meier, D.E., 118
memory, 79–80
Mental Health Systems Act of 1980, 119
Merleau-Ponty, M., 96
methodology, 13, 86
microaggresions, 7
Miles, S.H., 29
moral capacity, 8
morality, 114, 115
Morse, J.M., 11

N
Nakayama, T.K., 83
narrative, 79–80, 92, 105
National Commission for the Protection of Human Subjects, 29, 31
National Council on Aging, 103
Neumann, F., 6
Ngunjiri, C., 95
Nuremberg Code, 30
Nuremberg trials, 30

O
objectification, 63, 119
Olson, H.C., 118
Omnibus Budget Reconciliation Act of 1980, 119
ontological suppositions, 8, 114
ontology, 13, 86–87, 103, 114
Orbe, M.P., 83

P
Padmanabhan, S., 6
participatory theory, 103
Paxton, B., 95
Paying for Senior Care, 55
Pennebaker, J.W., 96
Perkins, P., 53
personal support system, *65*, 67
phenomenology, 1, 5, 8, 9–10
    agony, 92–96
    autoethnography and, 11–13, 85–92, 103
    data collection and, 83
    life journaling and, 83

Phinney, J.S., 82
Pick, A., 51
Pick's disease, 51
Plassman, B.L., 52, 53
Plato, 115
Pollock, F., 6
Poth, C.N., 13, 86
power vulnerability, 36
pragmatic meanings, 12
pragmatism, 6
Prairie View A&M University, 17, 18, 19
primary progressive aphasia (PPA), 51
psychosis, 56
Ptahhotep, 114
Pulling, B.W., 118

Q
qualitative research, 8

R
Rabaca, R., 6
Rabins, P., 58
race, 82
racism, 7
Râmbu, N., 121
Reagan, R., 119
Reason, P., 103
reflective journaling, 95
relational dialectical theory, 83
Republic, 115
research
    African American participation in, 30–31, 36–37
    IRB and, 29–30
    typology of orientations, 42–43
Richardson, L., 84
Road Not Take, The, 84
Robinson-Riegler, B., 79
Robinson-Riegler, G.L., 79
Rocco, T.S., 63
Rohr, R., 95
Rubinstein, R.L., 37

S
sacred space, 95
Sample Proximity Schematic, 33
Scharff, D.P., 42
Schulz, R., 118
self-in-relation-to-others, 95
semantic dementia (SD), 51
Shillingford-Butler, A., 82
Situated Positional Intersectionality, 77, 78
Skloot, R., 37
slaves, 36–37
Smith, L.M., 80
social morality, 117
Socrates, 115
stairs, 104–6, 110–13
    continence issues and, 106–7
    recordings of descending, 108–9

Stefancic, J., 7
St. Pierre, E.A.S., 84
Strauss, A.L., 92
structuralism, 104
suffering, 12
Sullivan, S., 12
sundowning, 58
supererogation, 119–22

T
Tamas, S., 35, 38
Tang, M.X., 53
Teachings of Ptahhotep, The, 114
Teall, E.K., 29
Templer, J., 105
Thimsen, K., 118
Torrey, E.F., 119
triggers, 37
Tullis, J.A., 32, 34, 38
Tuskegee Study, 30–31, 37

U
universal design, 68
University of Texas, 15
unspeakable, 97
unwritten reminders, 78
U.S. Public Health Service, 30

V
Vacation Bible School (VBS), 4
Vagle, M.D., 90, 91
Valois, L., 61, 63, 68, 118
van Manen, M., 11, 83, 97

W
Waldrop, D., 118
Washington, H.A., 30, 36
We Wear the Mask, 38
Weil, F., 6
White privilege, 7
White racism, 7
Whitinui, P., 81
Wilkerson, I., 17
Winau, R., 29
Wise, T., 7
Woodson, C.G., 7
World Medical Association, 30
written reminders, 78
Wycoff, S.M., 82

Y
Yeo, G., 51, 53
Yu, D.S.F., 7, 8

Z
Zahavi, D., 85
Zuckerman, M., 82